The Simple Guide to Revenue Cycle Hiring

The Simple Guide to Revenue Cycle Hiring

PENNY M. CROW

M. CHRISTINE KALISH

SHARON Z. GINCHANSKY

MGMA

Medical Group Management Association®

Item: 1022

ISBN: 978-1-56829-685-2

Printed in the United States of America

10 9 8 7 6 5 4 3 2 1

Contents

Purpose of the Hiring Guide

"People are not your most important asset. The right people are." – Jim Collins

The Basics

This book will help you think about hiring in ways you haven't thought about it before. Throughout this book, you will see small icons that will indicate three categories of information.:

	General information that is repeated in each of the hiring guides published by MGMA
	Specific information that is required information for the category of jobs being discussed and is only in this manual.
	These are isolated boxes meant to highlight information like pro tips and best practices.
	Key takeaway summaries are included throughout.

The core information in this guide is focused on the full recruitment cycle, outlined below:

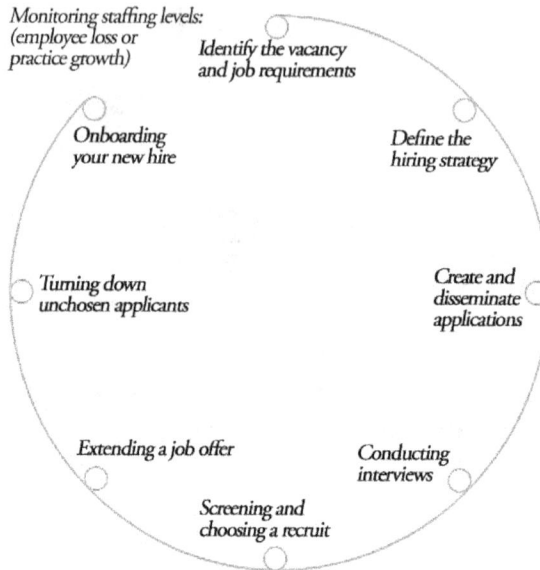

Monitoring staffing levels: (employee loss or practice growth)

Identify the vacancy and job requirements

Onboarding your new hire

Define the hiring strategy

Turning down unchosen applicants

Create and disseminate applications

Extending a job offer

Conducting interviews

Screening and choosing a recruit

Why does a medical practice need a hiring guide?

For many practices, hiring and recruitment is not a full-time, or even regular, activity. This hiring guide is written for everyone who manages staff or might be responsible for tasks involving human resources. This can be a narrow or broad group of resources and can include practice managers, physician-owners, and other staff, such as supervisors, recruiters, interviewers, trainers, compensation managers, HR specialists, legal/compliance coordinators, and researchers.

This guide takes the reader through the entire process from job analysis to description creation and through to hiring and onboarding. While it includes documents, tools, and related job descriptions, the guide is written in such a way that a practice can reference a certain section to focus in on just that information. This manual is tactical and process-oriented, providing step by step instructions for hiring tasks that might not be included in the daily workstream. It outlines the proactive strategies required to define, attract, and retain qualified applicants.

One of the challenges in a medical practice, especially smaller ones with limited resources, is the limited preparation before a vacancy occurs. When the manager receives a two-week notice from someone considered to be a valued or key employee, a couple of things tend to occur. First, the manager thinks they have more time than really exists to replace that employee; second, the manager imagines they might be able to convince the employee to stay. The reality is that the manager must act, and act quickly. Without a clear-cut process that can be immediately executed to begin the recruitment process, the gap for the practice may have nearly-immediate impacts on day-to-day operations. This manual, when used to its maximum benefit, will assist the medical practice in building a base for recruiting, hiring, and retaining staff that will allow the responsiveness and quick pivots required for today's medical practice environment.

This guide addresses the consistent processes and points out those that are specific to the job category in the title. While the rules and regulations for hiring and recruiting may be similar, different job levels and categories present unique challenges along the way. This tool provides tricks, tips, and best-practice ideas to support every size medical organization.

All staff should have access to this tool. Too often, organizations limit human resources and hiring functions to those who supervise, manage, or own the practice. Almost all staff, at one time or another, will be asked to participate in some part of the recruitment and hiring process. This guide also ensures *everyone* follows the appropriate process when bringing new staff into the practice. Additionally, this guide may help employees understand how their job relates to others in the practice. Sharing this information, so employees understand cause and effect, job performance, and the importance of improvement, benefits the entire organization.

Analyzing Medical Practice Staffing

"Time spent on hiring is time well spent." – Robert Half

As much as an organization wants to think that they are proactive about planning for staff changes, too often those plans are set aside when faced with the clear priority to provide excellent care to patients and deliver the associated day-to-day tasks. When a vacancy opens within an organization, the natural inclination is to move forward with filling the position as quickly as possible. The better strategy is to use the vacancy as an opportunity to assess staffing needs and determine if the organization can benefit from doing more than just hiring for the same job. This activity will take more time, but what the practice will gain in the long run by having a well-rounded team cannot be underestimated.

Even before the practice writes or updates a job description, the manager needs to make sure the projected position will meet the needs of the organization. Asking some questions and completing a short analysis will set the baseline for the hiring process and define an order of operations.

The first step is to better understand why there is an opening. What caused the individual to leave the position?

Reasons can include:

- Workload
  - Real or perceived workload disparities will create disagreements in the practice.
- Personality and fit
  - Company culture can make or break a team, and team attitude can make or break the culture.
- Managerial issues
  - People don't leave jobs; they leave managers.
- Compensation
  - Real or perceived compensation discrepancies create disgruntled employees.
- Training
  - A practice cannot expect the best from employees if they aren't trained appropriately.
- Personal
  - Life events and family commitments that are out of the practice's control.
- Career Advancement
  - It is difficult to provide numerous advancement opportunities in a smaller practice, however, there are different methods of addressing that in order to retain employees.

The practice can determine the answer to these questions through employee interviews and exit interviews—and through observing workflow and the personal interactions. There are tools available to model the process. The key is to keep this simple.

Depending on the answer to the above question, focus on different analyses to determine reasonable changes. Realistically, some things cannot be changed, but the practice may be able to balance that out with the issues that can be changed. For example, if this is about workload, analyze the staffing changes that can be made so the workloads can be distributed more equally and effectively. Small practices are challenged because staff may fill several roles. Roles can grow organically because a staff member may be a stellar performer and won't say no to the extra workload. This easily occurs when services are added that only require a few hours a week, such as scheduling for a part-time provider. The challenge is that workload can grow exponentially and eventually become unmanageable, creating employee dissatisfaction.

Job analysis is usually designed to be work-oriented or worker-oriented. A *work-oriented analysis* results in specific tasks being identified in a typical workday. For example, the receptionist in a small practice may answer phones, schedule appointments, collect monies, and balance the cash drawer. An example of a work-oriented result would be: 'It's time to convert to an electronic process rather than doing a task manually.' A *worker-oriented analysis* focuses on the qualities of the employee, such as knowledge, skills, abilities, and other characteristics (KSAOs) that will contribute to an employee's success in the job.

> A **work-oriented analysis** results in specific tasks being identified in a typical workday. A **worker-oriented analysis** consists of identifying the knowledge, skills, abilities, and other personal attributes that will be important to your practice. It is easier to teach how to complete tasks than it is to make someone fit your culture. Knowing exactly what is needed in a person will make it clearer to identify and hire toward.

Although it is important to hire competent staff, it is equally important that the competent staff also have emotional intelligence, empathy, communication, and other soft skills. This guide discusses how to identify these skills through interviewing techniques. Making poor hiring decisions costs money, creates liability, and results in lost time. Using best practices mitigates these risks. For example, the receptionist needs to be friendly, detail-oriented, reliable, and trustworthy. Whatever job analysis format you use,make sure you are consistent when writing all job descriptions. This information can also be used to determine the salary for a position, training needs, and the performance management process for feedback and evaluation.

Reviewing Relevant Regulations

Before getting into the specifics of the job, it is important to be aware of employment laws that may affect your individual positions. The section below is taken from MGMA's *Job Description Manual for Medical Practices*, 4th Edition (2019).

FLSA (1938)

The **Fair Labor Standards Act of 1938 (FLSA)**, as amended, established minimum wages, equal pay, and overtime; outlawed child labor; and specified record-keeping affecting most full- and part-time employees. One critical part of the law spotlighted in job descriptions is the designation of "exempt" or "nonexempt" job classifications. *Exempt* means that employees holding these jobs are not eligible for overtime pay. These are primarily professional positions. For example, if registered by the state, nurses meet the learned professional exemption and may be classified as exempt if paid on a salary basis of at least $455 per week. Nonexempt employees, such as clerks, are eligible for overtime when they work more than 12 hours in a workday or if they work more than 40 hours in a workweek. The Department of Labor designates which jobs are in which category. The designations do change occasionally. Supervisors should work with an HR specialist to make sure they know which positions are exempt or nonexempt and what that means in terms of overtime pay and other factors.

EPA (1963)

The **Equal Pay Act of 1963 (EPA)** applies to all employers covered by the federal wage and hour law under the Fair Labor Standards Act (see below). It requires that men and women be given equal pay for equal work in the same establishment. The job content, as described in the job description, determines whether jobs are substantially equal.

OSH Act (1970)

The **Occupational Safety and Health Act of 1970 (OSH Act)** established regulations to provide for the health and safety of employees on the job and the Occupational Safety and Health Administration (OSHA). The Act aims to ensure better working conditions by establishing guidelines for employers and employees on work environment conditions. The section in a job description titled "work environment" is a response to this Act and must consider such environmental factors as lighting, workspace, and identifying hazards. Employers must document, track, and report occupational injury and illness trends. Every medical practice should have a safety training plan and conduct such training during orientation and at regular times during employment. Examples of training include courses on body mechanics, infection control, and biohazard protection.

EEO (1972)

The **Equal Employment Opportunity Act of 1972**, referred to as **EEO**, extends the anti-discrimination provisions of Title VII of the 1964 Civil Rights Act. Your lawyer and an HR specialist can help ensure your job descriptions, hiring, and other employment practices comply with the mandate that individuals must be protected against employment discrimination on the basis of race, color, sex, national origin, and religion. It applies to employers with fifteen or more employees. There are two other legal issues to consider. When writing job descriptions, list only the minimum necessary requirements such as education and experience. It is acceptable to note preferred or desirable additional factors, but the emphasis must be on those that are necessary to ensure members of minority groups are not artificially screened out. Also, job descriptions should not state that a job can only be performed by a licensed professional when that is not actually a requirement of the state. For example, states require RNs to be licensed; however, medical assistants are not required to be licensed.

ADA (1990)

The **Americans with Disabilities Act of 1990 (ADA)** prohibits private employers, state and local governments, employment agencies, and labor unions from discriminating against qualified individuals with disabilities in job application procedures, hiring, firing, advancement, compensation, job training, and other aspects of employment. The ADA covers employers with fifteen or more employees. The Act does not protect every disabled person. The person also must be qualified, i.e., an individual who, with or without reasonable accommodation, can perform the essential functions of the job in question. The job description must clearly define those essential job responsibilities, the work environment, the equipment operated, the physical demands, as well as the required knowledge, skills, and abilities. Any person can then be compared with this job profile to ensure the qualification standard is met. HR specialists have the expertise to ensure that you comply with this critical legal regulation.

HIPAA (1996)

The **Health Insurance Portability and Accountability Act of 1996 (HIPAA)** not only focuses on accountability for ensuring patient privacy and confidentiality, it also protects the ability to continue to qualify for health insurance benefits if the employee changes or loses his or her job. It is the patient privacy and confidentiality piece that impacts a job description. Although job descriptions do not need to specify the "need-to-know" level of a job, they frequently emphasize the confidentiality requirement. In all cases, it is important for the supervisor to clearly define a job's confidentiality factors. For example, a clinician caring for a patient needs to know the person's diagnosis; a janitor in the facility does not.

HITECH (2009)

The **Health Information Technology for Economic and Clinical Health Act of 2009 (HITECH)** provides HHS with the authority to establish programs to improve healthcare quality, safety, and efficiency through the promotion of health IT, including electronic health records and private and secure electronic health information exchange. HITECH greatly impacts the need for technological proficiency.

Much of the listed legislation and regulation will affect the medical practice in some way.

Pro Tip: Keeping your eyes on the prize.

- Determine what skillsets can be taught and what must be brought to the table.
- Document the required skillsets.
- Determine traits.
- Determine what is the practice's responsibility to teach, remembering that training is not a one and done.
- Expand the touchpoints for finding competent candidates; this will help you resist the impulse to make the easy hire.
- Be aware that quickly-achieved, short-term relief will almost always equal long-term aggravation.
- Don't forget that it will tend to cost the practice from 3 to 5 times the annual salary if the hire is a mistake.

Conducting a Job Analysis

In larger practices, a consultant may be contracted to complete a job analysis. However, it isn't necessary to bring someone from the outside. The internal hiring manager can use the same tips and tricks for success. First, interview leadership to determine what expectations were set for the job. Next, interview the supervisor of that position, and then, finally, interview the person that actually does the job. It is always educational to see the disconnect between the three descriptions for the same position. This sort of job analysis can help address these discrepancies and provide a decision tool for what the roles and responsibilities of each job should be and, thereby, create a performance standard.

Another way to conduct a job analysis is to observe the current holder of the position and document the tasks being performed. Observing rather than interviewing allows a practice leader to determine if each of these tasks and processes are necessary for today's medical practice. Alternatively, some practices find it useful to have employees complete preprinted questionnaires. And last, but not least, other resources from MGMA may be appropriate for determining the specific tasks and KSAOs necessary for a job. It is important to document all essential functions of the job within the job description. Essential functions are what are considered when an employee requires accommodations made under the ADA. Questions to determine essential job functions include:

- Is this task truly necessary for the job?
- How often does this task have to be done?
- What percentage of time is spent doing this task?
- What happens if the employee doesn't do this task? (Are there consequences?)
- Can the tasks be done differently?
- Can the task be reassigned to someone else?

Now is the time to consider exactly what tasks the position is performing for the team and ask if those tasks:

- are necessary;
- add value; and
- support the core business, which is taking care of the patient.

In addition, consider if technology can be implemented or updated to relieve manual processes. You may find that the position is not really what you thought it was, and so making modifications may ensure retention in that position for the next candidate while boosting the productivity of the entire area or practice. Broken processes and incorrect staffing create significant inefficiencies and cost the practice in quality service, decreasing both patient and employee satisfaction.

If compensation is an issue, first look at the salary or hourly wage relative to the market. Market survey data is available through many sources to determine if the position is being compensated fairly for the work expected. Often this data is difficult to find, particularly when positions are identified differently by each practice. The front desk staff could be patient services representatives or medical receptionist, both doing the same job. When this happens, more analysis is required. Always look in your own backyard to determine if certain positions tend to move frequently, then consider other benefits to encourage retention. In all cases, re-evaluate the budget to see if there is room to increase the salary to be competitive and attract top candidates. Remember that a change for one equals a change for all. Adjusting compensation to keep one employee is never a good idea for the organization.

Take the time to step back and assess workflows to make sure the organizational structure is producing the optimal results. Ask yourself these questions:

- Are there inefficiencies that can be addressed?
- Are there processes that are broken?
- Are there reasons for all tasks being performed?

An individual new to the practice is not accustomed to doing things the usual way, so there is a great opportunity to map out process improvements that can be put into place with a fresh perspective.

Then, always consider personality and fit. Organizational culture, whether the practice is large or small, dictates employee and consequently, patient satisfaction. Be able to understand and communicate the company culture. Know if it's important to have a voice. That will help plan and focus your search. Know who and what you are hiring for.

Wrapping up: Analyzing Medical Practice Staffing

Taking the time to do a thorough analysis of your medical practice staffing is well worth the investment. Before leaping in to quickly replace a departing employee, make sure to gather all the information required to determine the correct staffing solution going forward for the practice. It is also imperative to make sure you understand the market for the role you do wish to hire and that your compensation package is competitive to acquire the quality staff the practice requires.

Key Takeaways

- Reconsider simply recycling the same job description to fill a new vacancy.

- Assess the reasons for the vacancy and make modifications as necessary to make the role as successful as possible.

- Go a step further and see if there are changes that can be made to current processes and workflows to make the organization perform at a higher level.

- Clearly understand your practice culture

Revenue Cycle Roles within the Medical Practice

> You hire the best people you can possibly find. Then it's up to you to create an environment where great people decide to stay and invest their time."—Rich Lesser

Undoubtedly healthcare is one of the most complex industries from both an operational and a financial perspective. There are few industries that interface with clients, patients, and stakeholders in the way that healthcare does while providing many different types of services. Medical practices are challenged in the current healthcare environment, experiencing a changing regulatory environment, reimbursement challenges, larger consumer payments, with shrinking margins for the medical practice. In addition, patients recognize the choices they have, including requests for transparency in all aspects of their care. Suddenly providers are faced with new challenges in consumerism, with patients focused on costs and insisting on increased quality of care. It is more difficult to maintain operating margins and deliver quality care. And practices are continually living in two worlds, balancing between the traditional reimbursement models while moving to value-based care. These drivers affect the entire practice, the entire revenue cycle.

The Healthcare Financial Management Association (HFMA) defines the revenue cycle as all administrative and clinical functions that contribute to the capture, management, and collection of patient service revenue. The term includes the entire life story of the patient experience from first contact to full account settlement. Functional areas of the revenue cycle include:

- Front-end roles: These are the patient-facing aspects of the cycle, including pre-visit and point of service functions.
- Mid-cycle roles: These are charge capture, coding, and submission functions.
- Back-end roles: These focus on billing, claims, and collections functions.

This tends to be an easy way to describe processes and discuss tasks. However, the revenue cycle includes all organizational layers, providers, staff, and management, and all processes related to their functions. Everyone is involved in patient engagement, performance, and productivity, and therefore the revenue cycle. Staff that fall under the revenue cycle job category will start with patient contact with the scheduler and progress all the way through the process to the financial analyst who produces the monthly reports. This hiring guide will

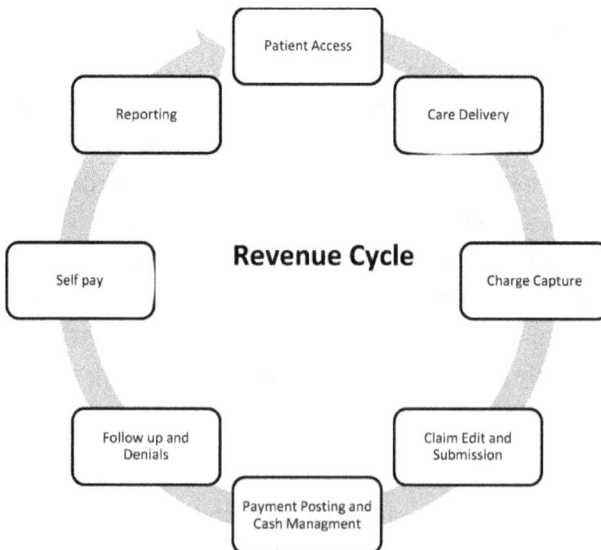

provide a broad view of revenue cycle job descriptions and focus on those positions that have historically been back-end functions.

The revenue cycle team is expected to take the data provided to them from patient visits, ensure the data is entered into the practice management system appropriately, and track the billing and reimbursement process until the claims are paid. They are expected to:

- Interact with patient access to reconcile the patient activity.
- Correctly post payments.
- Work the claims rejections and denials.
- Reconcile accounts and payments.
- Ensure accounts are reimbursed appropriately.

However, these tasks can be performed more efficiently if those members of the team that engage in the front-end tasks complete their work accurately. This means by entering the right data, such as patient demographics and insurance information correctly the first time and also verifying the information regularly. The earlier in the revenue cycle incorrect data flows, the harder and more costly it is to fix it.

The job descriptions in this category may include:

- Claims Analyst
- Collections Agent
- Medical Billing/Coding Specialist
- Medicare Coordinator
- Reimbursement Specialist
- Coders

However, it is important to include:

- Scheduler
- Front Desk Clerk
- Health Information Management (HIM) Technician
- Financial Analyst
- Office Manager

In smaller practices, the revenue cycle functions can be managed by one or two people. Staff will function in different roles or combinations of roles depending on the needs of the practice. This guide focuses on the recruitment, hiring, and retention processes for these core positions, identifying those candidates best qualified to serve in these roles.

The patient role is unlike other customers. They are in a vulnerable position as they seek medical care, when the challenges can be significant. It becomes difficult to gather the correct information in order to properly serve the patient. That's why it's so important to understand the skills and attributes needed for the revenue cycle positions. This guide will include the most detail for claims analysts, billing and coding specialists, insurance coordinators, reimbursement specialists, and collections staff.

The skillsets are as broad as the jobs in the revenue cycle. The skill commonalities include:

- Excellent customer service skills,
- Problem-solving abilities,
- Great attention to detail,
- Critical thinking skills,
- Open to change and technology, and
- Emotional intelligence.

Let's break this category into specific roles and consider the skills, competencies, and characteristics that will make a potential candidate successful in that job function.

Billing and Coding Specialists

Responsibilities and skills could include:

- Thorough knowledge of data collection and entry
- Coding and clinical documentation
- Substantial knowledge of medical bills, insurance payments, and policies with point of service collections
- Robust knowledge of HIPAA and privacy practices
- Specialty-specific coding expertise

Their competencies include:

- In-depth understanding of coding and billing procedures, often specialty-specific.
- Taking care to identify the patient correctly.
- Completing insurance verification.
- Providing financial counseling, if necessary.
- Identifying and delivering patient service recovery opportunities.
- Staying current with coding certifications.

Some of the success characteristics include:

- Substantial experience in healthcare and patient management
- Service- oriented demeanor
- Excellent communication skills
- Good understanding of math
- Attention to detail
- Technologically savvy

The ability to communicate difficult payer concepts to patients and their families is incredibly important for success in this role. There's a saying, "If it's not documented, it didn't happen." Coders are often responsible for working with providers to ensure the documentation matches the services provided so that they can reconcile the patient encounter with the assigned codes so the practice can be paid appropriately for services.

Claims Analysts

This is the partner role to the charge capture and billing. Responsibilities and skills could include:

- Monitoring charges and verifying correct payment of claims.
- Working denials, which includes sending appeal letters and tracking responses.

- Researching and resolving claim problems.
- Preparing reimbursement analysis by payer.

Their competencies include:

- Understanding HIPAA and privacy practices well enough to direct their conversation and provide answers.
- Acquiring deep knowledge of clinic policies and procedures.
- Understanding the information required for insurance verification and billing.
- Understanding different types of insurance and plans.

There is significant overlap in the success characteristics for the claims analysts and the billing and coding specialists. In both instances, the staff in those positions will be successful if they have:

- Substantial experience in healthcare and patient management
- Service- oriented demeanor
- Excellent communication skills
- Good understanding of math
- Attention to detail

Front Desk Clerk

The National Association of Healthcare Access Managers, (NAHAM), reported that about 80 cents of every dollar entering a healthcare facility goes through the hands of staff who are dually categorized as patient-access services and revenue cycle staff. The first encounter patients have in this role will be the front desk staff. Their competence lies in their ability to juggle different stakeholders and tasks at one time. Responsibilities and skills could include:

- Providing excellent customer service.
- Thorough data collection and entry.
- Coding and clinical documentation.
- Coordinating care, including referrals and scheduling other healthcare visits.

- Substantial knowledge of medical bills, insurance payments, and policies with point of service collections,
- Robust knowledge of HIPAA and privacy practices.
- Money management skills.
- Understanding of release of information.

Their competencies include:

- Answering the phone promptly with minimal dropped calls.
- Reducing hold time for callers.
- Answering with a pleasant demeanor.
- Understanding HIPAA and privacy practices to appropriately direct their conversation and answers.
- Scheduling appointments correctly and with the appropriate urgency.
- Coordinating communication within the practice.
- Being organized.
- Understanding the information required for insurance verification and billing.

Some of the success characteristics include:

- Outgoing personality,
- Easy-going disposition,
- Able to think quickly from call to call,
- Deep knowledge of insurance plans and services,
- Extreme attention to detail,
- Ability to interact with all types of stakeholders and personalities,
- Pleasant voice, and
- Helpful attitude.

The ability to communicate in different modalities with compassion and understanding is key skillset for success in this role.

Wrapping up: Revenue Cycle Roles

This chapter is a simplistic orientation to the revenue-cycle job category within medical practices. A more thorough listing of revenue cycle job descriptions is provided in Appendix A. It takes all these related positions to document, reconcile, and protect revenue cycle functions within a medical practice. The complexity of the systems and processes and the integration require significant oversight with strategically placed checks and balances. No matter the size of the practice, well placed and trained staff will protect the interests and sustainability of the organization and the patient. Now that you have a grasp on analyzing staffing and where patient-access roles fit into the medical practice structure, the next chapter will walk through the steps to create a job description.

Key Takeaways

- Soft skills and emotional intelligence are key to successful employees in the clinical job category.

- These positions focus on delivering care while integrating the implications from federal, state, and local regulations.

- Continuing education to keep up with current knowledge and trends in their specialty is generally a requirement for these positions.

Preparing the Job Description

"Under conditions of complexity, not only are checklists a help, they are required for success."—Atul Gawande

Once the cause of the vacancy has been analyzed, it is necessary to determine if the job description is still valid. A job description is a necessary tool that explains how the tasks and duties of a specific job fit into the practice's overall mission and strategic goals. It is important to keep job descriptions up to date, but there is no better time to reassess a position than when it is, or is about to be, vacant.

Writing the Job Description

All job descriptions within the practice should look the same. Standardization and consistency are two of the best defenses in human resource management. Job description methodology continues to be the safest way for employers to have documentation that supports employment decisions and avoids legal issues and complications in hiring, training, and terminating staff. Most importantly, a job description's primary purpose remains stable: to clearly communicate how the employee helps fulfill the goals of the organization. One way to write a job description is to answer the following questions. These answers will design a best-practice-formatted job description. Below are the seventeen core questions to be answered about the position.

Below each question in a gray box is an illustrative (not comprehensive) example response.

1. What is the job title?

- Make the title reflect what the job does. Not only is it important for the employee to understand the title, but a patient reading a name tag needs to be able to determine what this person does. Keeping it simple is always the best naming convention, so be cautious about being creative with titles. Simplicity is one of the best communication tools for the employee and patients to understand the role.

> **Job title:** Office Manager

2. What is the job classification?

- The Fair Labor Standards (FLSA) is very specific regarding exempt vs. non-exempt positions. *Non-exempt* means that you must pay overtime. Conversely, an *exempt* role is one that is management- or leadership-focused and oversees other staff. Know your state laws and the legal requirements to determine if overtime will be paid on daily or weekly work hours over the standard eight-hour workday. Many practices want to save money by making all their clinical positions exempt to prevent overtime, but the level of responsibility is a primary consideration of job classification. When in doubt, consult an HR professional or attorney for clarification. This conservative approach will protect the practice and the employee from violating IRS rules.

> **Job classification:** Exempt

3. To whom does this position report?

- This should list the title of the person they will be their supervisor. Keep in mind that the CEO or owner may still report to a board of directors, partners, or investors.
- Dotted lines between multiple supervisors is not recommended.

> **Reports to:** Practice Owner

4. When was the job description last reviewed?

- It is helpful to make sure the job is still relevant by dating the job description, which can help trigger a re-assessment if enough time has passed. Nothing can hurt a new employee's satisfaction faster than having the wrong expectations for the job. It is particularly important for executive positions to determine the scope of work executive and the level of expertise needed from the very beginning.

> **Date:** 08.01.2019

5. What is the summary of the overall job duties?

- This is a summary that allows an employee or candidate to quickly know the expectations.

> **Summary:** A management position responsible for the daily operations of the medical practice.

6. What are the essential job responsibilities for this position?

- It is important from an employment law defense perspective that essential job responsibilities are listed to determine the applicability of ADA accommodations. The employee will need to be able to successfully complete these specific responsibilities with reasonable accommodations.

- These are the tasks that regardless of physical or mental ability must be done in this individual job.

Essential Job Responsibilities:

- Ensure compliance with current healthcare regulations, medical laws, federal and state laws, and high ethical standards.
- Oversee daily office operations and delegate authority to assigned supervisors.
- Assist supervisors in developing and implementing short- and long-term work plans and objectives for clerical functions.
- Develop guidelines for prioritizing work activities, evaluating effectiveness, and modifying activities as necessary. Ensure that office is staffed appropriately.
- Assist in the recruiting, hiring, orientation, development, and evaluation of clerical staff.
- Establish and maintain an efficient and responsive patient flow system.
- Oversee and approve office supply inventory, ensure that mail is opened and processed, and offices are opened and closed according to procedures.
- Support and uphold established practice policies, procedures, objectives, quality improvement, safety, environmental and infection control, and codes and requirements of accreditation and regulatory agencies.

---

7. What are the competencies (KSAOs) needed?

- It is important for the practice and potential candidate to assess if they are a good fit for each other. This is only possible if the competencies (KSAO) are identified in advance.

• Describe the personal attributes that this employee must have to be successful in this role.

Competencies:

Knowledge

- Knowledge of policies and procedures to manage operations and ensure effective patient care.
- Knowledge of the principles and practices of healthcare administration, fiscal management, and government regulationsand reimbursements.
- Knowledge of Electronic Health Systems.
- Knowledge of Practice Management Systems.
- Knowledge of medical practices, terminology, and reimbursement policies.
- This position requires strong working knowledge of managed care plans, insurance carriers, referrals, and precertification procedures.

Skills

- Skill in exercising a high degree of initiative, judgment, and discretion.
- Skill in analyzing situations accurately and taking effective action.
- Skill in establishing and maintaining effective working relationships.
- Skill in organizing work, delegating and achieving goals and objectives.
- Skill in exercising judgment and discretion in developing, interpreting, and implementing departmental policies and procedures.
- Mastery of spoken and written English.

- Additional languages preferred.
- Possess strong human relations, communication, problem solving, and organizational skills to interact with a variety of customers, payers, vendors, and personnel within and outside the institution.

Abilities:

- Ability to work under pressure, communicate, and present information.
- Ability to read, interpret, and apply clinic policies and procedures.
- Ability to identify problems, recommend solutions, and organize and analyze information.
- Ability to establish priorities and coordinate work activities.
- Ability to work independently and be goal-directed.
- Effectively multitask without compromising quality.
- Ability to comprehend and excel in both verbal and written communication, including proper telephone
- Ability to communicate with individuals and small groups with credibility and confidence.

Other:

- Willingness and desire to maintain regular and acceptable attendance; may be required to work weekend, holiday, or overtime hours.
- Willingness and drive to handle complex, difficult interactions, remain calm under stress, manage emotional situations, display empathy, and maintain positive communication within a rapidly changing/ dynamic environment.

8. Are there any supervisory responsibilities?

- Not all people are leaders and teachers. Supervisory responsibilities include both those attributes. The practice can protect itself by establishing supervision expectations from the beginning. Identify any direct reports.

> **Direct reports:** Business Office Manager, Facilities Manager, Administrative Assistant, Receptionist.

9. What equipment is does the job require?

- Anything that may affect the employee's working conditions such as climate, noise, hours, construction.

> **Equipment:** Employee expected to be able to use standard office equipment, including computers, fax machines, copiers, printers, telephones, etc.

10. What is the work environment?

- Anything that may affect the employee's working conditions such as climate, noise, hours, construction.

> **Work environment:** Employee works in a collaborative medical office environment with a private office for confidential conversations. Moderate noise (i.e. business office with computers, phone, and printers, light traffic). Ability to work in a confined area. Ability to sit at a computer terminal for an extended period of time.

11. What are the physical and mental demands of the essential job functions?

- Identify any lifting, bending, sitting, standing, vision, hearing, dexterity and driving requirements.
- Also include any expected mental demands.

> **Physical and mental demands:**
> - Involves sitting approximately 90% of the day, walking or standing the remainder.
> - Combination of sitting, standing, bending, light lifting and walking.
> - Requires a full range of body motion, including manual and finger dexterity and hand-eye coordination.
> - Lifting up to 20 pounds.
> - Requires corrected vision and hearing to a normal range.
> - Occasional stress from varying demands.

12. **Is this a full time or part time job?**

   - Identify the typical work shift, days and overtime expectations

> **Position type and expected works hours:** Full time, business hours, Monday through Friday, but occasional evening, holiday, and weekend work. Some flexibility required. Must be available to have a mixed schedule of opening and closing the office and the ability to be flexible with schedule when needed.

13. **Is travel involved?**

   - Candidates need to understand if they are required to travel between clinic locations. Policies will need to be written to outline reimbursement guidelines.
   - List percentage of travel time expected, where the travel occurs, and whether it is overnight travel.

> **Travel:** Limited travel, primarily local during business hours. Less than 10% of monthly hours.

14. What is the required education and experience?

- Indicate education based on requirements that are job-related and consistent with business necessity. Remember, job descriptions should not state that a job can only be performed by a licensed or certified professional when that is not actually a requirement of the state.

Required Education and Experience:

- Bachelor's degree.
- Individuals may also need to complete additional coursework upon hire.
- Completion of a medical terminology course, or successfully completing one within six months of employment.

---

15. What is the preferred education and experience?

- Indicate preferred education and experience, but it must relate to this job specifically

---

Preferred Education and Experience:

- College-level coursework in healthcare administration preferred.
- Minimum three years of administrative experience, including at least one year of management experience in healthcare

---

16. What other eligibility qualifications exist?

- List additional licensure or certification necessary to have this job.

Additional eligibility qualifications:

- MGMA or PAHCOM certification.

---

17. What other duties as assigned?

- There is no way to identify every task in a practice. This is a general disclaimer statement that catches any other assigned duties.

> Please note this job description is not designed to cover or contain a comprehensive listing of activities, duties or responsibilities that are required of the employee for this job. Duties, responsibilities, and activities may change at any time with or without notice.

18. Include two signature lines.

- The employee and hiring manager should sign the job description and date it.

Putting It All Together

Now that you've answered these questions, you have all the components required to create the final job description. A sample job description for an office manager has been created. Keep in mind this is to be used an an illustrative guide only. This job description and all job descriptions provided in this hiring manual will need to be edited to describe the specific requirements your organization has for that role. Include any information that helps make the duties, responsibilities, and expectations for the role clear.

Job title: Office Manager
Classification: Exempt Reports to Practice Owner Reviewed: 08.01.2019

Summary:
A management position responsible for the daily operations of the medical practice.

Essential Job Responsibilities:

- Enhance patient experiences; optimizing company reputation.
- Ensure compliance with current healthcare regulations, medical laws, federal
  and state laws, and high ethical standards.
- Oversee daily office operations and delegate authority to assigned supervisors.
- Assist supervisors in developing and implementing short- and long-term work plans and objectives for clerical functions.
- Assist supervisors in understanding/implementing clinic policies and procedures.
- Develop guidelines for prioritizing work activities, evaluating effectiveness, and modifying activities as necessary. Ensure that office is staffed appropriately.
- Assist in the recruiting, hiring, orientation, development, and evaluation of clerical staff.
- Establish and maintain an efficient and responsive patient flow system.
- Oversee and approve office supply inventory, ensure that mail is opened and processed, and offices are opened and closed according to procedures.
- Support and uphold established policies, procedures, objectives, quality improvement, safety, environmental and infection control, and codes and requirements of accreditation and regulatory agencies.

Competencies:

Knowledge

- Knowledge of policies and procedures to manage operations and ensure effective patient care.
- Knowledge of the principles and practices of healthcare administration, fiscal management, and government regulations and reimbursements.
- Knowledge of Electronic Health Systems.
- Knowledge of Practice Management Systems.
- Knowledge of medical practices, terminology, and reimbursement policies.
- This position requires strong working knowledge of managed care plans, insurance carriers, referrals, and precertification procedures.

Job title: Office Manager

Skills

- Skill in exercising a high degree of initiative, judgment, and discretion.
- Skill in analyzing situations accurately and taking effective action.
- Skill in establishing and maintaining effective working relationships.
- Skill in organizing work, delegating and achieving goals and objectives.
- Skill in exercising judgment and discretion in developing, interpreting, and implementing departmental policies and procedures.
- Skill in planning and supervising.
- Skill in evaluating the effectiveness of existing methods and procedures.
- Mastery of spoken and written English;

Abilities

- Ability to establish and maintain effective working relationships with other employees and the public.
- Ability to communicate and present information under pressure.
- Ability to read, interpret, and apply clinic policies and procedures.
- Ability to identify problems, recommend solutions, organize and analyze information.
- Ability to establish priorities and coordinate work activities.
- Ability to work independently and be goal-directed.
- Effectively multitask without compromising quality.
- Ability to comprehend and excel in both verbal and written communication,
  including proper telephone etiquette, face-to-face interactions, and electronic
  communications.
- Ability to communicate with individuals and small groups with credibility and confidence.

Other

- Willingness and desire to maintain regular and acceptable attendance; may be required to work weekend, holiday, or overtime hours. Must be available to have a mixed schedule of opening and closing the office and the ability to be flexible with schedule when needed.
- Willingness and drive to handle complex, difficult interactions, remain calm under stress, manage emotional situations, display empathy, and maintain positive communication within a rapidly changing/dynamic environment.

Position Type and Expected Works Hours:

Full time, business hours, Monday through Friday, but occasional evening, holiday, and weekend work. Some flexibility required.

Job title: Office Manager

Equipment Operated:

Standard office equipment, including computers, fax machines, copiers, printers, telephones, etc.

Physical and Mental Demands

- Involves sitting approximately 90% of the day, walking or standing the remainder.
- Combination of sitting, standing, bending, light lifting and walking.
- Requires a full range of body motion including manual and finger dexterity and hand-eye coordination.
- Lifting up to 20 pounds.
- Requires corrected vision and hearing to a normal range.
- Occasional stress from varying demands.

Travel:

- No travel is expected for this position.

Required Education and Experience:

- Bachelor's degree,
- Individuals may also need to complete additional coursework upon hire.
- Completion of a medical terminology course or successful completion within six months of employment.

Preferred Education and Experience:

- College-level coursework in healthcare administration preferred.
- At least one year of healthcare administration experience.

Additional Eligibility Qualifications:

- MGMA, PMI, or PAHCOM certification.

Other Duties:

Please note this job description is not designed to cover or contain a comprehensive listing of activities, duties or responsibilities that are required of the employee for this job. Duties, responsibilities and activities may change at any time with or without notice.

Signatures

This job description has been approved by all levels of management:

Manager_____

Employee signature below constitutes employee's understanding of the requirements, essential functions and duties of the position.

Employee_____ Date _____

Wrapping up: Preparing the Job Description

This Office Manager job description is simply a road map. A carefully constructed job description identifies what is negotiable and what isn't for this clinical function. When this important stage of hiring is overlooked, it is much easier to compromise what is needed for the position, which can result in a poor hiring decision. Making poor hiring decisions costs the practice money, creates liability, and results in lost time. Using best practices will mitigate these risks.

It is as important for the candidate to assess the practice as vice versa. A well-written job description can be the perfect communication tool. Although the interview is important for a face to face discussion, it is the job description that is setting the tone for the discussion. It is also one of the best defense tools in employment complaints.

The job description helps ensure that the future employee and the practice are a good fit for each other. It sets the expectations from the beginning and can be used for orientation, feedback sessions, and the annual performance review. A good job description protects both the employer and the employee from unexpected surprises.

So, what's next? It is time to recruit to find the right candidate for the right job.

Key Takeaways

- Job descriptions should complement the practice mission.
- Good job descriptions establish the expectations of the candidate, employee, and management.
- It is necessary to know key HR laws when writing job descriptions to protect the practice.

The Recruitment Process Reconsidered

"Hiring the best is your most important task."
Steve Jobs

Recruitment at its core, is a basic, fundamental activity in all businesses. It is a process that if done well will help secure the practice's future. Why is it so important? It's important because it helps solidify the practice's reputation.

Consider this—if you walked into a medical practice for an interview, the front desk was unmanned, they weren't aware you were coming in for an interview, the interview was then conducted haphazardly and unfinished, what would you walk away thinking about that medical practice? Most likely, you would walk away thinking the practice does not know what they are doing, they were disorganized, disorderly, and treated you poorly.

How would you talk about that practice in the future? You, and others, would speak ill of the practice, telling this story possibly years to come. This might just be an interview gone awry and may not be a clear picture of the practice, but the story would linger in a negative way.

How do you rectify this? Using best practices to recruit staff that create the workplace culture you want in your medical practice. If you have recruited properly and filled your open positions with the best fit from a business and culture perspective, your business will thrive.

Satisfied employees create a satisfied patient population, which will create a successful practice, according to studies reported by *Forbes*. A successful practice means there is a likelihood that the practice will continue. Business continuity and continuation is vital, without successful caring individuals who think of your business as their business, your practice won't reach its full potential. This impacts not only the sustainability of your practice but the growth and the revenue overall. Your employees are your first line of customer service, excellent customer service will bring your patients and families back time and again.

The Recruitment Process

The recruitment process, from analysis to onboarding, is a costly endeavor. The process takes time and energy to complete in a manner that acquires the best candidates and the best employee. The costs associated with recruitment are extensive, including the time it takes away from your core business, but it is a requirement.[1] In a series of case studies analyzed by the Center for American Progress, it was found that 'quick hiring' could save an employer up to 50% of the employee's annual salary versus a full recruitment drive with analysis—but that there would be a better than 25% chance that within a year employee turnover would cost the company anywhere from 5% up to 213% of the employee's annual salary.[2] This is why hiring has to be executed well the first time around. Besides the financial deterrent associated with recruiting and hiring the wrong employee, there are other impacts that will ripple through your entire business in a number of ways—some that cannot be calculated, including:

- decreased productivity,
- turnover,

---

[1] Bersin, Josh. "Employee Retention Now a Big Issue: Why the Tide has Turned," LinkedIn Influencer, August 16, 2013, https://www.linkedin.com/pulse/20130816200159-131079-employee-retention-now-a-big-issue-why-the-tide-has-turned/

[2] Boushey, Heather and Sarah Jane Glynn. "There Are Significant Business Costs to Replacing Employees," Center for American Progress, November 16, 2012, https://www.americanprogress.org/wp-content/uploads/2012/11/CostofTurnover.pdf

- decreased patients seen,
- delayed service times,
- negative viewpoints from customers and employees,
- not enough resources,
- lower morale,
- gossip, and
- information not shared between staff.

The only way to mitigate these costs is hire right the first time using tried and true methods to bring in the best candidate.

What is your turnover rate?

How many people left your practice last year? (X)

What were the total number of positions last year? (Y)

Divide number who left by the number of positions. (X/Y)

That's your turnover rate—for every role turned over, there is both a replacement cost and a cost to your business for not having that role filled

---

How to start the recruitment process.

After you have completed the analysis and determined your practice's needs, consider both *how* and *where* to recruit.

How will you recruit for this position?

The simplest answer is that recruitment comes from many sources to attract and satisfy diverse candidates. It can also be described as using any way possible that yields the best candidates. Examples of methods include:

- Create a superior hiring package:
  - Offer better compensation than the local market.
  - Offer better benefits (such as health or 401K).
  - Offer better career advancement packages.

- Create a stronger culture fit:
  - Offer a closer knit, more supportive environment.
  - Offer a greater scope of employment-based interests and challenges.
  - Offer ties to the local community.
- Create a better tomorrow:
  - Offer education support.
  - Offer vested interest in the company.
  - Extend expanded benefits (not just health) to include employee families (a matching college fund for kids is a powerful retention tool for top recruits.)
- Create personal satisfaction:
  - Offer challenges tailored to the personality of the recruit.
  - Offer team-based reverse interviews to allow top recruits to "interview" you.
  - Allow for flexibility by allowing the recruit choice in one or more non-key functions (things like local charity drive management or inter-office sports activities).

CAUTION

Using a recruiter or a headhunter is expensive. It can cost in excess of 20% of the annual salary unless you have a retained agreement for the recruiter. Before you hire a recruiter, consider whether or not you can successfully recruit internally.

Where should I recruit from?

There are many places to garner qualified and experienced candidates. The first step is to determine if are you going to recruit for this position yourself without using an agency or a recruiter. If you choose to use a recruiter for this position, confirm the details of the contract. The contract should list and explain the associated costs, such as who has the responsibility to pay for any possible advertising or related out-of-pocket expenses. In addition, the contract should cover

Pro Tip: Ask your current employees for referrals, encourage them to seek out the candidates. Your employees know your workplace, they are well connected, they are your greatest recruiters. For tough to fill roles, incentivize employees with referral bonuses or raffles. Encourage them to post on their social media accounts.

what happens if a candidate applies for the position on their own and is also presented by the recruiter and how to manage previous candidates you've interviewed. It should also address how long the contract period is in place and identify the specific positions for recruitment. Then negotiate who completes the background or licensure verification and references and who your practice works with during the process. These items should be clearly delineated in the contract so you are not haggling or reviewing this after you've found your ideal candidate.

Finding the right candidate on your own is not only possible, but achievable, if you put in the effort. Start by thinking where you want to post the job opening.

The greatest asset you have is your current employee base. Begin by telling your employees the practice has a job opening, then give them a flyer or show them the job posting. Ask your staff for help to fill this job. Be clear with your employees what it is you're looking for in a potential candidate. The more direct you are with your staff, the better the referral will be in the long run. If you need someone who has a specialized degree, tell them. There is nothing worse than having someone referring be told after the fact you were looking for something specific. Don't let your employees put themselves out there with their colleagues or friends only to be embarrassed.

Pro Tip: Look at postings by searching the job title and seeing what others post. This will help you create the best post using keywords and common themes.

Posting an open position is relatively easy now with many little-to-no-cost options. As in all searches, the practice should have a plan to attract the most qualified candidates. Consider postings based on the position, as follows:

- **Create a job posting flyer.** List the who, what, where, when, how, and why of interesting tidbits the candidate will be searching for in their category. Make it appealing, eye catching, and easy to read.
- **Post to job boards like Indeed or ZipRecruiter.** Job boards have low cost models to help small businesses. Indeed also searches for web posts and will link to your job some of the time. Do not count on this, as it does not always happen.
- **Post to LinkedIn.** If your business does not have a LinkedIn account, consider this the ultimate time to start one. Moreover, create one for your practice administrator specifically to post these positions.

Where do you post for the job opening?

- Executive search firms will contact you—make adecision if you wish to do this, if not then proceed with normal recruitment activities .
- Networking—business contacts, community organizations (Rotary Club, Executive Coaches), former business associates.
- Indeed, ZipRecruiter, LinkedIn, Craig's List, local community colleges, local universities/colleges,
- Never underestimate the power of social media and personal relationships for these positions

Pro Tip: When posting for the job, if you want to an easy pre-screen, provide the requirements, such as a certification from HFMA or a CPA.

- **Social media.** Is the practice on social media? If so, use the flyer to post this position with a hyperlink for an email or application process.
- **Local schools.** Local universities and/or colleges are an excellent place to connect with job prospects. Alert the career center and/or professors/teachers in this field that you are hiring.
- **Your website.** This is a great place to sell your own organization. Your patients may have referrals and that will speak volumes about your practice!
- **Networking, local organizations, and affiliations.** Are you a member of local organizations or networking group? Do you attend monthly meetings in your field? These are logical places to post these positions and discuss the opening.

You have candidates, now who do you interview?

Most importantly, you must assess the candidates fairly.

- What should you be looking for?
  - Credentials
    - Be fair and equal—it is important to review all candidates equally to avoid any future concerns.
    - Minimum standards—candidates that do not meet the minimum standards will not be prioritied for interviews.
    - Preferred requirements—if applicants meet the preferred requirements, they will be placed at the top of the list for interviews.
    - Skills required for the position—if an applicant meets all the requested skills, the candidate will go to the top for interviews.
  - Job history
    - Assure the job history reflects the skills need for the posted position. It is important to inquire about gaps in the history.

- ○ Instructions
  - ❏ Did the applicant follow instructions properly on how to apply? For example, if you requested a salary history and he/she did not provide one, will you exclude the applicant? Perhaps not, but it is good to know your boundaries and what you're willing to waive. This is very important, because if you waive any for one applicant, you must waive it for all.
- ○ Résumé
  - ❏ Was the résumé tailored for your position? If it is a generic résumé, does it meet your needs?
- ○ Initiative
  - ❏ Did the applicant take initiative by reaching out to the hiring manager or practice administrator?
- ○ Cover letter
  - ❏ Did they send one? Is it specific to the job you are posting?

Pro Tip: Create a form to add on top of each résumé to assess each candidate fairly.

Include the following information:

- Candidate Name
- Position Applied For
- Date
- Minimum requirements listed
- Minimum requirements met
- LVN licensed
- CPR certified
- Bilingual
- Interview date

- o Results-oriented
  - ❑ Are the résumé results oriented to showcase their achievements or is it simply a history? This showcases the applicant's work ethic and interest in success.
- o Growth
  - ❑ Is there a history of being moved up, quick growth, or long history of growth? Is the candidate using your practice for growth or to find a home?
- o Competitor
  - ❑ Do they work for a competitor? If so, perhaps you want to interview to get a clearer understanding of the competitor's landscape.

The Application Process

You have now narrowed down your top candidates to interview. The final step in the recruitment process is having an application process that will help you and the candidate carefully discern if offering the position and having it accepted is the right choice for everyone. To best do that, you need to make sure you have an application process that gathers all the pertinent information required.

Do you need an application and a résumé for each applicant?

Absolutely, yes. The résumé is different from an application. The application is a legal document that includes a variety of items that showcase a chronological history of work history, education and skills. Before you interview the candidate, you must have information on each applicant for legal purposes. A résumé is something you will want to have, but it is imperative to have the candidate complete an application.

This is a two-part step that helps the practice get information standardized. All résumés are different and unique to help a candidate stand out to the employer. The application is an equalizer, so all candidates will be judged equally. It gives information about the applicant's background that is not on the résumé. Moreover, the application requires a signature at the end, acknowledging various legal aspects of the interview process. The process allows for more protection for the practice as well.

How do you create an application?

If the practice has a computer-based applicant tracking program, there is a good chance there is an online application process associated with it. Check your system and provider to determine if this is an option. If it is not, there are many samples on the internet to create your own application. The key components[3] to include are as follows:

- Practice name, address, and phone number or use company letterhead
- Applicant's legal name, address, phone number, and email
- Are you eligible to work in the United States? Yes | No
- Are you at least 18 years or older? (If no, you may be required to provide authorization to work.) Yes | No
- Have you ever been terminated from employment or asked to resign by an employer? Yes | No
  - *If yes,* please provide company names and details
- Work History (chronological order with start and end dates) with supervisor name and contact phone number or email along with reason left the employment
- Criminal history
- Salary history
- Educational background
- Preferred schedule (give specific boxes with available day/time combinations)
- How did you hear about us? Walk In | Advertisement | Referral | Other
- Have you ever worked for this company before?
- Do you know anyone who works for our company?
- Reference Listing (3) name, phone number, email, company

---

[3] Society for Human Resource Management (SHRM) example

- Legal signatures (signing that they understand the practice is an at-will employer)
- It is very important to include something like the following disclosure statement, which the applicant should sign separately:

Please read carefully before signing.

[Practice Name] is an equal opportunity employer. [Practice Name] does not discriminate in employment on account of race, color, religion, national origin, citizenship status, ancestry, age, sex (including sexual harassment), sexual orientation, marital status, physical or mental disability, military status or unfavorable discharge from military service.

I understand that neither the completion of this application nor any other part of my consideration for employment establishes any obligation for [Practice Name] to hire me. If I am hired, I understand that either [Practice Name] or I can terminate my employment at any time and for any reason, with or without cause and without prior notice. I understand that no representative of [Practice Name] has the authority to make any assurance to the contrary.

I attest with my signature below that I have given to [Practice Name] true and complete information on this application. No requested information has been concealed. I authorize [Practice Name] to contact references provided for employment reference checks. If any information I have provided is untrue, or if I have concealed material information, I understand that this will constitute cause for the denial of employment or immediate dismissal.

Date _____ Signature _____

THIS APPLICATION IS VALID ONLY FOR 60 DAYS FROM THE DATE SIGNED/DATED ABOVE.

Wrapping up: Recruitment

Mindful recruitment strategies will be one of the most important commitments you can make to growing the future of your practice culture, teams, and organization. Find ways to introduce consistency into your approach and maximize the potential of your networks and connections. An improved recruitment process can be one of those opportunities where a practice can reap the rewards a seasoned practice manager's persistence and dedication can bring to a problem.

> **Key Takeaways**
>
> - Being consistent in your approach and methodical in your processes will significantly benefit you and your practice or organization in the long run.
> - Careful preparation will help you hire the correct candidate.
> - A careful application process is the best way to make the seeds of your recruitment efforts bear fruit.

Designing a Hiring Process

"You don't hire for skills, hire for attitude. You can always teach skills." – Simon Sinek

After all the upfront time and energy you took to prepare for the recruitment and application processes, it is time to find the right candidate through a carefully crafted hiring process. This process has a series of fundamental steps, which will be outlined below. By implementing a few best practices, you will be able to refine your process and find the right candidate for your practice.

The Hiring Process

Keep in mind, as you build out your hiring process, that the first and foremost concern is to create a candidate experience that is positive. Aside from any damage the practice's reputation might suffer from word getting around about a poor interview experience, your ideal result is a candidate who very much wants to work for your practice. A carefully crafted process will provide the required structure when the impacts of day-to-day operations might normally cause you to forward in ways that are not ideal.

There will be some steps that will need to be altered depending upon the role being filled. One of those steps is the candidate interview. It can be helpful to have a pre-determined strategy for different types of roles, so that when you have an opening for that type of role, you are clear about your intended interviewing strategy. Similarly, having a pool of questions for those interviews available based on the role will help shorten the time required to prepare for interviews. See Appendix B for some suggested questions based on roles outlined in this hiring manual. Here is a broad outline of the hiring process:

1. Ensure that an applicant tracking system is in place and being followed.

2. Select an interview strategy if one is not already in place.

3. Identify important questions.

4. Prepare the total compensation calculation.

5. Outline ways to understand candidates' alignment with the practice culture.

6. Conduct phone and face-to-face interviews prioritized by candidates who are the best fit for the identified role requirements.

7. Make an offer.

8. Perform pre-employment requirement checks.

9. Communicate with declined applicants.

10. Onboard the new hire.

11. Have a process for reviewing the new hire during the probationary period.

Tracking System for Applicant Information

Most small practices and even larger ones will not have a tracking mechanism or system for tracking the applicants. Some payroll systems have this built in, so make sure to check with your payroll provider. If you don't have an automated system, an Excel spreadsheet is the easiest way track. If you don't have an Excel spreadsheet, you can create something similar in Word or by hand. The spreadsheet/document should include the applicant's name, application date, referred by, interview dates, including any phone interviews. If you have a much larger practice, you may want to invest in an applicant flow tracking system that tracks

> **Pro Tip:** Retain all applicant information collected and any related hiring notes for a minimum of 3 years.
>
> Preserve the application information for candidates within a personnel file in a locked filed cabinet behind a locking office door. Personnel file retention regulations vary from state-to-state, so check local/state laws for requirements.

applicants anonymously to help ensure no discrimination has taken place. You will also want to have an organized system for keeping all documents related to the hiring process in a secure location.

No matter how well you think it went, you still might receive a call from the EEOC (Equal Employment Opportunity Commission), the Department of Fair Employment and Housing (DFEH), or directly from a lawyer. This is where having your tracking and documentation in place as you go into the process will help you afterwards. Keep in mind, however, that it is not unusual for the EEOC or DFEH simply to be confirming information they have received. Or they may have an anonymous tip that the practice discriminates against a particular group. This is the moment when you take a *deep breath*, grab your hiring notes, your references, any information you pulled, whatever you did to interview and ultimately fill the position. Anything related from the general period of time when you hired that position should be your focus as you prepare to respond to the complaint.

If you receive a formal complaint, contact an HR consultant or a lawyer before answering the complaint. Time is of the essence. While this may be scary or nerve-wracking, do not delay, as there are specific timeframes for response associated with any complaint.

Considerations for small practices vs large practices

The information needed during a governmental review or if a lawsuit should arise is no different. The size of the organization will only come into play in order to determine if your practice is required to meet additional employment standards. The first magic number is 50; the second is 100. If you have fewer than 50 employees, there is some leeway with the requirements of employment laws. However, you must still treat every applicant with respect and dignity, no matter the size of your practice.

Select the Interviewing Strategy

First, determine the best approach to the interview for the particular role that is being filled. Interview strategies are not a one-size-fits-all decision. Some things to consider to select an interviewing strategy:

Who participates in the interviews?

The default choices tend to be the hiring manager or an HR specialist. Some practices opt to have a couple of interviews with different focuses: an HR specialist narrows down the field, then the hiring manager, then a peer or team member. Another alternative to consider would be a team-based approach. Particularly when roles are tightly embedded in a team-based, collaborative culture, the greatest way to accomplish a successful hire is a group interview. These can offer great insight about the team, the role, and the candidate.

Provide the interviewing team with the job description and meet with them to develop the agenda for the interview and an agreed-upon list of questions. Particularly for staff who have little experience interviewing candidates, thinking through the role, what sort of questions to ask, and who should ask them can help them think more thoroughly about what sort of skills and traits they should be looking for in the interview. It will also give you an opportunity to inform them about appropriate interviewing standards and techniques, and confirm the proposed questions conform to best practices (see the "Formulate the Questions" section of this chapter).

Adding a new team member to any group, can be a stressful and time-consuming. Ensure that the candidate's personality, communication style, and mannerisms will fit with the existing staff. Be cautious that individual nuances are not disguising discrimination but

Pro Tip: A phone screening can be a more casual interview; however, there should always be a specific list of questions to structure the interview and provide ease of comparison. Those questions can include:

- Where have you worked?
- Why are you interested in working for our practice?
- What type of job title, work schedule, and salary are you looking for in this role?
- What is prompting the search for a new role?
- When can you start?
- What would you say was your proudest work accomplishment?
- Do you have any questions I can answer?

Phone interviews will usually last from 15 to 30 minutes, depending on the role.

do ensure that the candidate is a complement to the existing staff and is the best fit for your patients. There should be enough similarities that colleagues have things in common, but not so much similarity that the practice loses the benefit of diversity. Team interviews are a great way to experience this fit and discern if the desired synergy is observed.

Use phone interviews to screen applicants

Always complete a phone interview before inviting candidates to your office. An in-person interview takes time, perhaps time that is not available since there is an opening. Conducting a phone interview allows the hiring manager or HR specialist to get a feel for the candidate before committing the time and resourcces to a face-to-face interview. It also allows the for the opportunity to rank applicants to guide the decision on who to invite for the in-person appointments. Phone interviews should be quick confirmations of basic details and a short information-gathering session in order to decide about inviting for an interview. If you've conducted the phone screening and you're not sure if the applicant should come in, let the candidate know you'll be in touch at a later date as you determine the interview schedules.

Take full advantage of the in-person interview

Creating a workplace interview that is positive is similar to creating a practice a patient will want to visit. Below is a possible scenario for setting up the interview for success:

- Invite the applicant to sit down and provide someplace they can wait comfortably. If there is going to be a delay that is any longer than 10 minutes, explain why and thank them for waiting.
- Offer a beverage.
- Provide the candidate with an interview schedule.
- You body language should be relaxed yet energetic. If you are busy and harried, the applicant will feel unwanted or an imposition.
- Treat the candidate respectfully with:
    o Direct eye contact
    o A firm handshake
    o A warm , welcoming smile
- When you invite the applicant into the interview room, make it clear where he or she should sit.
- Give the applicant a tour of the facility, which is an exercise that is useful to you and the applicant, as it is an opportunity to gauge how they fit in the practice environment.)

Formulate the Questions

You will want to prepare a number of questions in advance. Keeping a core list of questions you ask each applicant will ensure uniformity and make later comparisons more equitable. Consider asking behavior-

Pro Tip: There are a few simple best practices for face-to-face interview.

- Do *not* write on the applicant's résumé or application; use a pre-filled out paper to attach to the résumé/application.
- Give applicants a tour of the practice. Look for social or normal cues to determine if they have solid customer service skills and will be a good steward for the organization (e.g., o they make eye contact with the employees and with the patients. Do they pick up trash in the hallway? Do they converse while walking them around? Do they stop for conversation with people?)
- In an interview, it is okay for you to be quiet. Allow the applicant to add more to your question and their answer. If their answer is short, encourage them to tell you more.

based questions that can show you the character of candidates: how they will work and integrate into the culture of the practice. The key is to get to an understanding of how a possible candidate will relate to and solve situations with patients and other staff. The best practice for interviewing is to ask open-ended, conversational questions.

A sampling of open-ended questions includes:

- Please tell me about your career and your background.
- What do you know about this practice?
- What makes you the right candidate for this role?
- After walking the practice, what immediately would you want to change?

Some example scenario-based and behavior-based questions

- Tell me about difficulties you experienced in your last position.
- Describe what work environment makes you your most successful.
- What would you change about your last work environment?
- What do you want me to remember about you after this interview?
- Is there anything else I should know about you and your work history or possible work here?

The questions to never, never ask . . . ever

There are many questions that are inappropriate and unlawful to ask while in an interview. Generally, these are questions that pertain to a person's protected class. A protected class is a group of people qualified for special protection by a law, policy, or similar authority. Overall, it is best to avoid questions that are about gender, color, religion, national origin, gender identity, sexual orientation, political affiliation, family status, disability, or the like. These are questions that, if asked, may open up potential for a discriminatory filing or lawsuit.

A sampling of questions that you should **not ask** are listed below. This is **not** a comprehensive list.

DO NOT ASK
Are you married?
Do you plan to have kids?
What does your spouse do?
Where did you grow up?
What year were you born?
Do you have any bankruptcies?
Have you ever filed a worker's compensation claim?
Have you been injured at work before?
Do you normally wear your hair that way?

DO NOT ASK
Do you have a cane you will use when at the office?
How will you manage the wheelchair in the hallway?
If you got the job, how do you get to work?
Who did you vote for?
Are you a Republican or a Democrat?

Things to share about the practice

The interview process is not only a time for the practice to learn about the candidate, it is also a good time to make sure the candidate understands things about practice and organization standards, policies, and procedures. For example, some clinics don't pay mileage if the person travels straight from their home to the alternate clinic but will pay the standard reimbursement rate if change in location occurs during the day. This expectation should be communicated with the candidate during the interviewing stage. Anything that might be an unpleasant surprise on either side including restrictions on paid time off around holidays, dress code standards, or any other concerns the practice has had to manage in the past should be shared. Keeping a list of these items and sharing them with all applicants will protect the practice from the risk of complaints or litigation.

You've Made a Decision

You've done all the hard work and invested considerable effort into finding just the right person for the role and you now have a candidate you would like to bring onto the team. Now what? It is important at this point for the practice to follow the same hiring practices for each new hire, no matter the role. Implementing a few best-practices steps can go a long way in protecting the practice and providing the candidate the fair and equal opportunity they deserve. You may be eager to go ahead and extend an offer and close the deal, but make all final employment decisions contingent upon your all due-diligence verifications, including background checks, OIG clearance, drug screen, education verification, and skills checks.

Pro Tip: What to ask during a reference check:

- Verify candidate's employment dates, title, salary (they may not give to you).
- Ask if the person re-hirable.
- Ask for their overall impression of the candidate.
- Inquire if there is anything specific you should know about this candidate.

CAUTION: Making a hiring decision based purely on one person's reference-call responses could trigger a complaint if the candidate is not hired.

Reference Checks

It is a good idea to call the candidate's references before making an offer. The candidate should consent to you contacting at least three references. References should consist of former employers, supervisors, or colleagues. Reference questions should be standardized. You should ask each person the same questions and then document the answers in the same way. It is important to confirm dates of employment, job title, duties performed, and reason for separation. Remember that while a former employer can say anything that is factual and accurate, what qualifies as factual and accurate can be difficult to prove. Concern over lawsuits causes many former employers to only confirm position, attached salary, and the dates of employment. Despite this, always ask if there is anything they would like to specifically share with you about the candidate.

CAUTION: Do not disclose specific information the references shared with you if the reference is negative. This is confidential.

Document each call or email for the personnel file. Best practice is to have at least two references checked, previous employment or professional references. In some scenarios, a personal reference may be used, but this would be for an entry-level position or someone with little to no work experience. Whatever information is shared should be between you and the reference provider. It should not be shared with the candidate. Reference check are an excellent first line of defense that may protect your organization from having to endure the pain and costs of a bad hire.

Unfortunately, there are many candidates who are either blatantly dishonest or embellish the truth. It is important to fact check information presented by the candidate. You can use social media as a reference point; however, the practice should have policies around the use of this information. The policies will protect the organization, particularly if the social media research shows that the potential candidate belongs to a protected class. Under no circumstances can a person's class or right to free speech be violated or perceived to be violated in preventing them to be considered for a position. While it may be appealing to check on candidates to confirm they would represent your practice well on social media, unless your policies are explicit, acting upon this information may expose the practice to risks.

CAUTION:

Conducting any type of background check before a formal offer is made to the candidate is not appropriate. Do not ask candidates for any identity-related information (e.g., Social Security, previous names, aliases, etc.) without first making an offer.

Total Compensation

The explanation of compensation can be a difficult conversation, so be prepared before making an offer to paint this complete picture. Particularly if the applicant is in a role with labor pool shortages, it will be that much more important to explain the total compensation for the position. *Total compensation* includes all monies the employee will make in this role, including annualized salary, benefits, vacation time value, 401(k) investments, and educational benefits. This is the opportunity for the practice to show the prospective employee what they will fully earn during their employment on an annual basis.

This matters significantly to an employee, as it is their total picture of what they will earn, in salary as well as benefits. It may be useful for some practices to prepare a "Total Compensation Statement" they can provide to the employee to illustrate the true value of working for the practice. The more detailed information, the more beneficial it will be to the potential employee.

You may want to include the following items in a total compensation statement:

- Annualized pay
  - If position is hourly, take the hourly rate x 2080 to get this annualized number.
- Medical benefits
  - Include the amount paid by the employee *and* the employer contribution.
- Flexible spending account
  - Include details on how this is implemented.
- Paid leave
  - List all vacation/sick/PTO, holidays, personal days, floating holidays, or whatever else is offered.
- Volunteer opportunities
  - Describe the volunteer program and recent or near-future projects.
- Disability insurance
  - Short or long term
- Life insurance
  - If paid by the practice, show figures.
- Employee Assistance Program
- Educational Assistance or Tuition Reimbursement
  - Annual amount
- Retirement
  - 401(k) (include any matching).
- Career pathway or advancement

Offer Phone Call Example

Hello. This is _____ from _____. It was a pleasure meeting you and learning about you. After careful consideration we have decided we'd like to offer you the position of _____. The position would pay $_____ per hour, and we'd like you to start on _____. This offer is contingent upon you meeting a number of pre-employment requirements, including a drug screen, criminal background check, and education verification. If you are still interested in the position, we will send you an offer letter and will need some additional information.

Employment Offers and Offer Letters

Following satisfactory reference checks and a confirmed calculation of total compensation, you've reached the decision to extend an offer of employment. What is next? And how is it conducted? The simplest communication method and a best practice is to call the candidate directly and make a verbal offer.

Written offers of employment—contingent offers

The best practice for any type of employment offer, once a verbal offer is accepted, is to make a formal offer in writing. This is done in order to clarify what is being offered, what the pre-employment requirements are prior to the start date, and what the compensation, benefits, and perks for the position are. The letter should explain the offer is contingent upon satisfactory results returned for your practice's pre-employment requirements. The letter should also cover the hourly salary, paydays, supervisor information, benefit information, the start date(s) of those benefits, and who to contact for more benefits information. It should relay information about orientation, training details, schedule, and any other details that will help the new hire feel ready to go when they walk in the practice door on their first day.

Pre-employment Requirements

Every practice, no matter its size, should have a comprehensive list of pre-employment verifications that are performed before the hire is finalized. The practice will need to clearly communicate with the new hire that their employment offer is contingent on the results of those verifications.

Criminal background checks

Background checks are valubale source of protection for your organization. Although the process will cost money, it is minimal compared to what the unknown can cost. Candidates must consent to their background checks and provide their Social Security number, any previous names or aliases, and the names of counties that are applicable based on the candidate's previous residences. The general rule is to review the past 7 years of criminal history.

A reputable background check company should be able to advise you as to what your state/county/local ordinances allow for background checks. The company you have engaged should be able to guide you and recommend what is a best practice for your organization. If they are unsure or cannot provide what you believe to be credible information, move on to a new company. If you try using an internet search firm without customer service, you will most likely not get the type of background check that will satisfy the due diligence standards you and your practice would require. This type of search will yield simple and basic information that will not pass muster in a state or federal survey.

Pre-employment background checks must be administered in compliance with all federal, state, and local laws and all candidates must be treated equally. Decisions for employment cannot be based on a person's race, national origin, color, sex, religion, disability, genetic information, gender identity, ethnicity, political affiliation, or age. For more specific information, refer to the EEOC website.[1] Keep in mind that a criminal background does not automatically eliminate someone from a job. Make sure that you are not discriminating when considering this information. Sometimes the circumstances may influence your decision of the applicability of this information. If you are unsure about

---

[1] https://www.eeoc.gov/eeoc/publications/background_checks_employers.cfm

a candidate's background, it is best to seek out professional human resources consulting or legal advice.

Regardless of the background check results, treat the candidate with respect by keeping information private and confidential. This information is not intended to be shared with the general office population and should be kept in locked and secured files. This information should only be discarded by shredding the information and should not be disposed of in the regular waste basket. Just as a patient's information is considered private and confidential, the practice should protect any candidate and employee's private information.

HHS OIG clearance

Many background check companies will provide, as part of the standard healthcare background check, the U.S. Department of Health and Human Services Office of Inspector General (HHS OIG)'s listing to confirm the candidate is not on the List of Excluded Individuals/ Entities (LEIE), also known as *the exclusion list*. This is mandatory for clinical personnel and a choice for other personnel, however, best practice says conduct this check for all potential employees. The OIG has the authority to exclude individual from federally funded healthcare programs for a variety of reasons, including a conviction for fraud.[2] This includes any pending investigations being conducted by the OIG. If the background company you contract with does not do this, you must do this prior to day one, but after the contingent offer has been made. Any company or person who hires an individual on the list may be subject to civil monetary penalties. Complete this search yourself by visiting the OIG website as listed below and typing in the candidate's name. Take caution—many people have the same names; it is important to confirm identity when withdrawing a job offer.

Illicit drug screening

Many states require a pre-employment drug screen of all healthcare staff. Make sure to check local and state laws. Again, this is done post-

---

[2] https://oig.hhs.gov/exclusions/index.asp

offer and completed once an employment offer is made. Consent is required to conduct the pre-employment drug screen. Choose a vendor that specializes in pre-employment exams. It is best practice for the candidate to have one attempt for the urine drug screen. In other words, if candidates miss the scheduled appointment, they would automatically be disqualified as an employee of the organization.

Skills checks

If a specific skill has been identified in the job description, it is necessary to validate the information is true. This is precisely why a reference check is important. It gives an opportunity to confirm with a prior employer. If it is a new graduate, the instructor or a clinical site supervisor can be one of the references. If it is a technical skill or language competency, quizzes, assessments, or demonstration may provide the confirmation needed. This will be further reviewed in the section in the chapter on orientation and onboarding of personnel. A new hire will need to demonstrate competency in front of a supervisor or peer. This confirmation should be done prior to a new employee working independently without supervision.

Education, licensure, and certifications verification

All job offers should be made as contingent upon verification of education, licensure, and certification status. In recent years, news stories have reported that prestigious leaders of organizations have falsely claimed to hold degrees required for the positions they were holding. Unfortunately, it happens. To protect the organization, make sure to validate education, training, licensure, and/or certifications via the university, trade school, professional association, or state board conferring the credential. Ultimately, it is the leader's responsibility to ensure that the patients are being seen by qualified individuals.

It is essential to confirm all credentials after the offer, but prior to first day, in order to confirm the applicant's résumé is accurate. While you wouldn't expect a well-respected member of your community to not have an accurate résumé, you would be surprised by the percentage of people who do not put the correct information on their résumé. Confirming credentials differs for each role or position category. Larger organizations may use a service to confirm and validate, but smaller practices will usually complete it by phone or online. Either method works as long as it is completed and documented.

Specifically, for administrative positions, credentials may include:

- Degrees
  - Doctorate in business or public health
  - Master's degree in health services administration, business, public administration, health informaiton management, or public health
  - Bachelor's degree
- Licensure and credentials
  - CPA for accountants
  - SHRM for human resources managers
  - CMPE, CMM, CMOM certifications for practice managers
  - RHIA, RHIT certifications for health information professionals
- Published information or articles

What if the candidate does not meet the requirements?

Not all candidates will pass the pre-employment requirements. When this happens, it is challenging being the person who must rescind the job offer. The cleanest way to do this is to contact the candidate via phone and explain to them in a concise manner that the pre-employment requirements were not met. Tell them that you're very sorry, but you must rescind the offer, and you wish them the best of luck. Although the candidate will usually have some idea they have issues that might identified during pre-employment screening, it is not unusual for the candidate to nonetheless want specific information. If you utilize a company to complete the background check, you can refer them directly to that company. If you completed the background check yourself, you can share the information you discovered.

Occasionally, the information discovered during a pre-employment screening is false or unsubstantiated, e.g., the OIG has multiple similar names or perhaps the drug screen results are inconclusive. When there are questionable results from any of the pre-employment screening, it is recommended to contact the candidate and explain the situation. This gives candidates an opportunity to explain or rectify any issues identified. This is perfectly acceptable. The key is to provide a timeframe within which candidates must resolve the issues or discrepancies. Your position cannot remain open indefinitely. It is best to give the candidate a two-week period or 10 business days to resolve the issue or the offer is rescinded.

Declining other applicants

Many businesses fail to contact other interviewed candidates. It is a part of the process that no one, even the most skilled professional, wants to do. You are relaying a rejection to the candidate, which is difficult both to offer and receive. It is an uncomfortable but key part to closing out the hiring process. The best course of action is to contact each candidate via phone. The hiring manager or HR representative completing the search should contact the face-to-face candidates once the other candidate has passed all contingencies on their employment.

Onboarding Completes the Hiring Process

Onboarding is the time to bring the new employee into your organization, and it involves new hire orientation, training, and the probationary period. It is the opportunity not only to teach the job but

> **Pro Tip:** On an annual basis, all practice employees should be screened against the HHS OIG exclusion list, as this information does change. A suggested process is to run these names, print the results, and place them in a binder or a folder labeled "List of Excluded Individuals Screening for [YEAR]."

Pro Tip: Calculating the onboarding costs per hire

1. Total pre-employment screening costs per candidate .
2. Number of hours to orient and train multiplied by the hourly rate of the trainer
3. Number of hours to orient and train multiplied by the hourly rate of the new hire.
4. Advertising costs (if any)

Total re-employment screening costs = $85
Trainer time = $25 x 15 hours = $375
New hire time $15 x 15 hours = $225
Advertising costs = $75
Total = $760

This is an incredibly modest and conservative number.

to assimilate the new hire into the practice culture. This is the time to assess their skills hands-on and give them the opportunity to receive the benefit of having supervisor or peer training and guidance. Onboarding is the final piece of the puzzle to having a full-fledged successful member of your team. Proper onboarding is costly; it requires even more effort and time than recruitment. It may be tempting to reduce or eliminate it. But keep in mind that according to the Society for Human Resources Management (SHRM), 69% of employees are more likely to stay with a company for three years if they experienced great onboarding.[3] The majority of employees fail in the first 90-days of employment due to poor onboarding. A survey conducted by Allied Workforce Mobility discovered that companies lose 25% of all new employees within the first year.[4]

---

[3] Maurer, Roy. 2015, April 15. *Onboarding Key to Retaining, Engaging Talent.* Retrieved from https://www.shrm.org/resourcesandtools/hr-topics/talent-acquisition/pages/onboarding-key-retaining-engaging-talent.aspx.

[4] Allied Workforce Mobility Survey. 2012, March. Retrieved from http://hriq.allied.com/pdfs/AlliedWorkforceMobilitySurvey.pdf.

Make sure to have made all the arrangements and generated the necessary materials to properly onboard the new hire, including employee handbooks, training schedules, peer mentors information, before the new hire's first day. No one benefits from a last-minute scramble added to the already challenging practice environment. Take the time to discuss the onboarding process experience with employees once they complete the probationary stage and be prepared to implement improvements based on that feedback.

Probationary Period

A probationary period is the time the practice has determined is the training period required for the new employee to be successful in that role. A probationary period is generally 90-days. However, this does not mean you simply terminate the employee if they aren't doing a good job. That is not the intention of the probationary period. From day one of the probationary period, the practice should invest in training, assessing, and providing active feedback on the work product of the new employee. It is the supervisor's responsibility to accurately train and develop the new employee. The supervisor should supervise this employee by giving them the tools to be successful, answer questions, follow up on the day's work, and check in every day/week/month to assure the new employee understands and is completing their job assignments properly. The new employee should not at any time be wondering how they are doing in their new job; the supervisor must communicate this on at least a weekly basis, if not daily.

Be prepared for the new hire to struggle at points. It can be helpful to assign a peer mentor if possible or find another way to provide support.Not only will the new hire need support, but the staff will also be adjusting to a new teammate during this period.

Wrapping up: Hiring

The hiring process is the last chance for the candidate and the practice to determine mutual fit. Does the candidate fit the role as far as knowledge, skills, abilities, and attitude? Does the candidate fit with the team and practice culture? Is the role going to be the right one for the candidate?

Answering these key questions is pivotal to the success of the hire, the success of the team, and the success of the practice going forward.

Key Takeaways

- Create a positive candidate experience.
- There are many regulations around the hiring process. Be sure everyone involved has been educated on them, and the practices policies designed to mitigate risk. Don't hesitate to consult an HR specialist.
- Don't waste all the hiring effort by failing to properly train and onboard the new hire. A sink or swim philosophy is not goingn to create success for the new hire or the practice.

Summary

"Hiring people is a form of investing. You have to do your research and make sure you're spending your resources on the right pick."—Warren Buffett

The most important outcome of careful hiring processes is to have an employee base that shares the vision the leadership has for the practice. These employees will represent the practice for a long time. Keep the following points in mind:

- Treat everyone equally and fairly.
- Do not rush the hiring process.
- Prepare the new employee for success with a careful onboarding process.

Hopefully, hiring is not an everyday occurrence in your medical practice. But when it becomes necessary, this guide is available to help remind about best practices. In addition, it will help the practice be more prepared to place the right resources at the right time. Falling short in the hiring process will only lead to turnover in the position and may well have an effect throughout the entire organization. Healthcare is about delivering quality care to patients. Let's put the right people in the right place for the right reasons.

"Always treat your employees exactly as you want them to treat your best customers."—Stephen Covey

Appendix A:
Job Descriptions

Job Title: Claims Analyst

Department: Finance
Immediate Supervisor Title: Chief Financial Officer or Controller
Job Supervisory Responsibilities: None

General Summary:
- A non-clinical position responsible for the proper and timely processing of claims and payments to providers.

Essential Job Responsibilities:
- Oversees claim processing and payments to third-party providers.
- Answers associated correspondence.
- Monitors charges and verifies correct payment of claims and capitation deductions.
- Sends denial letters on claims and follows up on requests for information.
- Audits and reviews claim payments reports for accuracy and compliance.
- Researches and resolves claim and capitation problems.
- Ensure compliance with current healthcare regulations, medical laws, federal and state laws, and high ethical standards.
- Prepares claim reports for administration and finance on utilization and claim payment turnaround time. Identifies exceptional claims for review.
- Initiates payment recovery for stop loss reinsurance, worker's compensation, and overpaid claims.

Education:
- Bachelor's degree in health or business administration.

Experience:

- Minimum two years of experience in claims processing in a health care setting.

Competency Requirements:

Knowledge:

- Knowledge of clinic policies and procedures.
- Knowledge of health care insurance claim practices and compliance.
- Knowledge of computer systems, programs, and applications.
- Knowledge of medical terminology.

Skills:

- Skill in gathering and reporting claim information.
- Skill in trouble-shooting claim insurance problems.
- Skill in written and verbal communication and customer relations.

Abilities:

- Ability to work effectively with physicians, other medical staff, and
- external agencies.
- Ability to identify and analyze claim problems.

Equipment Operated:

- Standard office equipment including computers, fax machines, copiers, printers, telephones, etc.

Work Environment:

- Position is in a well-lit office environment. Occasional evening and weekend work.

Mental/Physical Requirements:

- Involves sitting approximately 90 percent of the day, walking or standing the remainder.
- Combination of sitting, standing, bending, light lifting and walking.
- Requires a full range of body motion including manual and finger dexterity and hand-eye coordination.
- Requires corrected vision and hearing to a normal range.
- Requires the ability to manage stressful situations.
- Occasional stress from varying demands.

Disclaimer: This description is intended to provide only basic guidelines for meeting job requirements. Responsibilities, knowledge, skills, abilities and working conditions may change as needs of the organization evolve.

Job Title: Collections Specialist

Department: Finance
Immediate Supervisor Title: Comptroller
Job Supervisory Responsibilities: None

General Summary:

- A non-clinical position responsible for collection of delinquent patient accounts.
- Corrects claims that are rejected from the claim's scrubber, clearinghouse or payer.
- Files secondary and tertiary claims as needed, electronically or via paper.
- Posts receipts from insurance companies and patients and edits any electronic remittance advice; may post from lockbox account on the web.
- May prepare deposits and/or make deposits.
- Generates patient statements.
- May check eligibility on patients with appointments and call patients whose insurance is not active .
- Calls patients who have not made payments in response to statements.
- May turn patients over to third-party collectors.
- Takes phone calls from payers or patients about billing issues and resolves issues.

Essential Job Responsibilities:

- Identifies delinquent accounts, aging period, and payment sources. Processes delinquent unpaid accounts by contacting patients and third-party reimbursors.
- Reviews accounts, credit reports, and other information sources such as credit bureaus via computer.
- Ensure compliance with current healthcare regulations, medical laws, federal and state laws, and high ethical standards.

- Performs various collection actions, including contacting patients by phone and resubmitting claims to third-party reimbursors.
- Evaluates patient financial status and establishes budget payment plans.
- Follows and reports status of delinquent accounts.
- Reviews accounts for possible assignment; makes recommendations to credit manager and prepares information for collection agency.
- Assigns uncollectible accounts to collection agency or attorney via clinic credit and collection policy.
- Contacts lawyers involved in third-party litigation.

Education:

- High school diploma or equivalent. Some college preferred.

Experience:

- Minimum two years of medical collections experience.

Competency Requirements:

Knowledge:

- Knowledge of medical billing/collection practices.
- Knowledge of basic medical coding and third-party operating procedures and practices.
- Knowledge of legal and regulatory government provisions.

Skills:

- Skill in establishing and maintaining effective internal and external working relationships.

Abilities:

- Ability to enter accurately data and examine insurance documents.

- Ability to deal courteously with patients, staff, and others.
- Ability to communicate effectively and clearly.

Equipment Operated:

- Standard office equipment including computers, fax machines, copiers, printers, telephones, etc.

Work Environment:

- Position is in a well-lit office environment. Occasional evening and weekend work.

Mental/Physical Requirements:

- Involves sitting approximately 90 percent of the day, walking or standing the remainder.
- Combination of sitting, standing, bending, light lifting and walking.
- Requires a full range of body motion including manual and finger dexterity and hand-eye coordination.
- Requires corrected vision and hearing to a normal range.
- Requires the ability to manage stressful situations.
- Occasional stress from varying demands.

Disclaimer: This description is intended to provide only basic guidelines for meeting job requirements. Responsibilities, knowledge, skills, abilities and working conditions may change as needs of the organization evolve.

Job Title: Medicare Billing and Coding specialist

Department: Administration

Immediate Supervisor Title: Office Manager,
Billing Manager, Comptroller

Job Supervisory Responsibilities: None

General Summary:

- Medicare Billing and Coding specialists work for healthcare facilities where they convert patients' information to standardized codes, which are used on documentation for Medicare insurance claims and for databases.
- Medicare Billing and Coding specialist assist practitioners to receive reimbursement from Medicare, and Medicare (Part c) plans.
- The Medicare Billing and Coding specialist will assign required Current Procedural Terminology (CPT), Healthcare Common Procedure Coding System (HCPCS), International Classification of Diseases, Tenth Revision, Clinical Modification (ICD-10-CM) and American Society of Anesthesiologists (ASA) codes.
- Assign Ambulatory Payment Classifications (APC) or Diagnosis-related group (DRG) codes.

Essential Job Responsibilities:

- Reviews notes from inpatient or outpatient encounters and codes them according to the documentation
- May post charges for services rendered.
- Audits chart documentation for quality purposes to ensure that provider coding and documentation is synchronous.
- Make judicious decisions on which codes to assign in each instance, and function to a high level of accuracy.

- Introduces changes in procedure (HCPCS) and diagnosis (ICD-10) codes and educates staff on the use of new codes.
- Ensures encounter forms and practice management software is updated appropriately with new and deleted codes.
- May be delegated the Compliance Officer.
- Liaising with physicians and other parties to clarify information.
- Examining documents for missing information.
- Assigning CPT, HCPCS, ICD-10-CM, and ASA codes.
- Assigning APC and DRG codes.
- Ensuring documents are grammatically correct and free from typing errors.
- Performing chart audits.
- Advising and training physicians and staff on medical coding.
- Informing supervisor of issues with equipment and computer program.
- Ensuring compliance with medical coding policies and guidelines.

Education:

- Certification in Medical coding for Medicare, Medicaid and Major Medical plans.
- High school diploma or GED and one year of customer service experience required, such as administrative, physician's office, appointment scheduler or retail/ service industry.
- Requires computer skills including Windows-based applications and intranet/internet use with the ability to keyboard and navigate through multiple applications.
- Individuals that have not completed a Medical Terminology course will be required to successfully complete a Medical Terminology course within six months of employment.

Additional qualifications:

- Associate degree and coursework in a healthcare related field is preferred (e.g., Administrative Clinic Assistant, Medical Office, Medical Assistant, Healthcare/Medical Receptionist or comparable).
- Must be AHIP qualified.
- Exposure to electronic health record preferred.
- Ability to work independently, be goal-directed and have strong organizational skills.
- Effectively multitask without compromising quality.
- Ability to comprehend and excel in both verbal and written communication, including proper telephone etiquette, face-to-face interactions, and electronic communications.
- Ability to communicate with individuals and small groups with credibility and confidence.
- Ability to handle difficult situations, remain calm under stress, manage emotional situations, display empathy and maintain positive communication during a rapidly changing/dynamic environment.
- Turn problems into opportunities by developing innovative and creative solutions.
- Demonstrate a friendly, positive attitude, display energy and drive in performing daily responsibilities.
- Must be flexible as well as easily adapt to a changing work environment which will require ongoing maintenance of job-related skills/activities.
- Must be willing to adjust work schedules in response to department or clinical needs.
- Able to manage and prioritize tasks simultaneously while working directly with patients who may exhibit diverse needs.
- Basic Life Support (BLS) may be required in some areas.
- Individuals may also need to complete additional coursework upon hire.

Experience:

- Minimum two years of administrative experience, including one year with a health care organization.
- [Medical specialty] office experience is a plus.

Other Requirements:

- Must be available to have a mixed schedule of opening and closing the office and the ability to be flexible with schedule when needed.

Competency Requirements:

Knowledge:

- Knowledge of and experience with [vendor-specific EHR] is preferred
- Knowledge of proper phone etiquette and phone handling skills
- Knowledge of organizational policies, procedures, and systems.
- Knowledge of office management techniques and practices.
- Knowledge of computer systems, programs, and applications.
- Knowledge of research methods and procedures sufficient to compile data and prepare reports.
- Knowledge of grammar, spelling, and punctuation.
- General knowledge of healthcare terminology preferred.
- Knowledge of purchasing, budgeting, and inventory control.

Skills:

- Skill in taking and transcribing dictation and in the operation of office equipment.
- Requires strong personal computer skills, communication skills, problem solving, continuous improvement and teaming skills.

- Maintains a broad knowledge of this practice's clinical, financial, and administrative systems/applications and processes.
- Demonstrated verbal and written communication skills.

Abilities:

- Must maintain regular and acceptable attendance; may be required to work weekend, holiday or OT hours.
- Ability to establish and maintain effective working relationships with other employees and the public.
- Ability to work under pressure, communicate and present information.
- Ability to read, interpret, and apply clinic policies and procedures.
- Ability to identify problems, recommend solutions, organize and analyze information.
- Ability to establish priorities and coordinate work activities.

Equipment Operated:

- Standard office equipment including computers, fax machines, copiers, printers, telephones, etc.

Work Environment:

- Position is in a well-lit office environment. Occasional evening and weekend work.

Mental/Physical Requirements:

- Involves sitting approximately 90 percent of the day, walking or standing the remainder.
- Combination of sitting, standing, bending, light lifting and walking.
- Requires a full range of body motion including manual and finger dexterity and hand-eye coordination.
- Requires corrected vision and hearing to a normal range.

- Requires the ability to manage stressful situations.
- Occasional stress from varying demands.

Disclaimer: This description is intended to provide only basic guidelines for meeting job requirements. Responsibilities, knowledge, skills, abilities and working conditions may change as needs of the organization evolve.

Job Title: Medicare Coordinator

Department: Finance
Immediate Supervisor Title: Chief Financial Officer or Controller
Job Supervisory Responsibilities:

General Summary:

- A position responsible for assisting with and monitoring the delivery of care and tracking for the Medicare populations.

Essential Job Responsibilities:

- Assists physicians and other providers in assessing the optimal level, type, and mix of medical care for Medicare patients.
- Enhance patient experiences; optimizing company reputation.
- Ensure compliance with current healthcare regulations, medical laws, federal and state laws, and high ethical standards.
- Oversees Medicare Quality Improvement initiatives, identifies quality of care deficits, and assists with developing interventions to ensure treatment.
- Coordinates geriatric disease management program; focuses on approaches to chronic illness while emphasizing efficiency and cost effectiveness.
- Participates in disease management programs and coordinated health care plan chart reviews of Medicare risk population.

Education:

- Bachelor's degree in nursing.
- AHIP Qualification.

Experience:
- Minimum three years of clinic and case management experience.
- [Specialty-specific] experience preferred.

Other Requirements:
- Must be available to have a mixed schedule of opening and closing the office and the ability to be flexible with schedule when needed.
- Licensed registered nurse.

Competency Requirements:

Knowledge:
- Knowledge of clinic policies and procedures.
- Knowledge of case management practices and compliance.
- Knowledge of Medicare government and insurance requirements.

Skills:
- Skill in gathering and analyzing Medicare information.
- Skill in troubleshooting Medicare problems and claims.
- Skill in written and verbal communication.

Abilities:
- Ability to work effectively with patients, physicians, and health plan representatives.
- Ability to identify and analyze quality care concerns.

Equipment Operated:
- Standard office equipment including computers, fax machines, copiers, printers, telephones, etc.

Work Environment:
- Position is in a well-lit office environment.
- Occasional evening and weekend work.

Mental/Physical Requirements:

- Involves sitting approximately 90 % of the day, walking or standing the remainder.
- Some bending, stooping, and lifting up to 25 pounds.

Disclaimer: This description is intended to provide only basic guidelines for meeting job requirements. Responsibilities, knowledge, skills, abilities and working conditions may change as needs of the organization evolve.

Job Title: Reimbursement Specialist
Department: Finance
Immediate Supervisor Title: Chief Financial Officer or Controller
Job Supervisory Responsibilities: None

General Summary:

- A position responsible for performing billings and collections for alpha, discipline, and/or payer.

Essential Job Responsibilities:

- Reviews all claims within designated alpha and discipline before claim release.
- Attaches required documentation to claims for payments.
- Assists customers with billing questions.
- Enhance patient experiences; optimizing company reputation.
- Ensure compliance with current healthcare regulations, medical laws, federal and state laws, and high ethical standards.
- Researches and corrects all denials received for designated alpha and discipline.
- Documents all correspondence with patients, insurance carriers, and vendors.

Education:

- High school diploma or equivalent. Some college preferred.

Experience:

- Minimum one year of medical billing experience.

Other Requirements:

- Must be available to have a mixed schedule of opening and closing the office and the ability to be flexible with schedule when needed.

Competency Requirements:

Knowledge:

- Knowledge of medical terminology.
- Knowledge of clinic policies and procedures.
- Knowledge of computer systems, programs, and spreadsheet applications.

Skills:

- Skill in oral and written communication.
- Skill in time management and organization.

Abilities:

- Ability to maintain confidentiality of all business/work information.
- Ability to effectively work with others.

Equipment Operated:

- Standard office equipment including computers, fax machines, copiers, printers, telephones, etc.

Work Environment:

- Position is in a well-lit office environment.
- Occasional evening and weekend work.

Mental/Physical Requirements:

- Involves sitting approximately 90 % of the day, walking or standing the remainder.
- Combination of sitting, standing, bending, light lifting and walking.

- Requires a full range of body motion including manual and finger dexterity and hand-eye coordination.
- Lifting up to 20 pounds.
- Requires corrected vision and hearing to a normal range.
- Requires the ability to manage stressful situations.
- Occasional stress from varying demands.

Disclaimer: This description is intended to provide only basic guidelines for meeting job requirements. Responsibilities, knowledge, skills, abilities and working conditions may change as needs of the organization evolve.

Job Title: Business Office Manager

Department: Administration
Immediate Supervisor Title: Chief Financial Officer
Job Supervisory Responsibilities: General
supervision over business office staff

General Summary:

- A management position responsible for directing and coordinating the overall functions of the business office to ensure maximization of cash flow while improving patient, physician, and other customer relations.

Essential Job Responsibilities:

- Reviews current status of patient accounts to identify and resolve billing and processing problems in a timely manner.
- Plans and directs registration, patient insurance, billing and collections, and data processing to ensure accurate patient billing and efficient account collection.
- Manages the business office within the established budget, including annual planning, and develops monthly status reports.
- Establishes and implements a system for the collection of delinquent accounts ensuring third-party payers are contacted.
- Establishes and recommends credit and collection policies.
- Makes recommendations for improvement.
- Maintains contacts with medical records and other departments to obtain and analyze additional patient information to document and process billings.
- Develops and oversees business systems and works with information technology to ensure timely and accurate implementation.

- Makes recommendations for improvement for all processes.

Education:

- Bachelor's degree, preferably in business administration or related field.

Experience:

- Minimum five years of experience in a medical business office, two years as a department manager in business office department.
- Other Requirements: None

Competency Requirements:

Knowledge:

- Knowledge of business management and basic accounting principles to direct the business office.
- Sufficient knowledge of policies and procedures to accurately answer questions from internal and external customers.
- Broad-based knowledge of relevant insurance regulations and familiarity with the Health Insurance Portability and Accountability Act.

Skills:

- Skill in establishing and maintaining effective working relationships with other employees, patients, organizations, and the public.
- Skill in developing, implementing, and administering budgets.

Abilities:

- Ability to communicate in writing, over the telephone, and in person with office staff and insurance representatives.

- Ability to recognize, evaluate, solve problems, and correct errors.
- Ability to conceptualize work flow, develop plans, and implement appropriate actions.

Equipment Operated:

- Standard office equipment including computers, fax machines, copiers, printers, telephones, etc.

Work Environment:

- Position is in a well-lit office environment. Occasional evening and weekend work.

Mental/Physical Requirements:

- Daily activity is 80 percent sitting and 20 percent walking or standing.

Disclaimer: This description is intended to provide only basic guidelines for meeting job requirements. Responsibilities, knowledge, skills, abilities and working conditions may change as needs of the organization evolve.

Job Title: Customer Service Specialist

Department: Marketing
Immediate Supervisor Title: : Marketing Manager
Job Supervisory Responsibilities:

General Summary:

- A position responsible for responding to and following through on customer inquiries, issues, and concerns in a timely and accurate manner.

Essential Job Responsibilities:

- Responds to telephone inquiries relating to the medical practice's policies and procedures.
- Facilitates patient visits and supports the health care provider by anticipating and responding to patient needs and requests of the health care team.
- Allows care providers to focus on patient care by coordinating details of patient visits, which can include; coordinating complex appointment schedules and daily activities of the care providers in a multispecialty medical practice, preparing patients, completing pre-examination record information, managing the flow of patient materials.
- Obtains or verifies patient demographics, medical insurance information, and properly advises patients of scheduling delays or changes to the appropriate individuals and serves as a direct contact and resource to the patient.
- Responds to written correspondence from customers.
- Researches customer complaints/concerns and takes appropriate actions to resolve them.
- Provides accurate information to customers regarding insurance benefits, providers, claims, referrals, eligibility, pharmaceuticals, etc.

- Properly documents and files all customer complaints and results.

Education:

- High school diploma or GED and one year of customer service experience required, such as administrative, physician's office, appointment scheduler or retail/ service industry.
- Associate degree and coursework in a healthcare related field is preferred (e.g., Administrative Clinic Assistant, Medical Office, Medical Assistant, Healthcare/Medical Receptionist or comparable).

Experience:

- Minimum three years of experience in customer service, preferably in the health care industry.

Other Requirements:

- Must be available to have a mixed schedule of opening and closing the office and the ability to be flexible with schedule when needed.

Competency Requirements:

Knowledge:

- Knowledge of medical terminology.
- Knowledge of insurance industry and billing procedures.
- Knowledge of grammar, spelling, and punctuation for written and verbal correspondence.

Skills:

- Skill in using computer programs and applications.
- Skill in conflict resolution.
- Skill in exercising a high degree of initiative, judgment, and discretion.

- Skill in analyzing situations accurately and taking effective action.
- Skill in establishing and maintaining effective working relationships.

Abilities:
- Ability to handle multiple priorities at the same time.
- Ability to read, understand, and follow oral and written instruction.
- Ability to communicate clearly and concisely.
- Ability to establish effective working relationships with patients, employees, and the public.

Equipment Operated:
- Standard office equipment including computers, fax machines, copiers, printers, telephones, etc.

Work Environment:
- Position is in a well-lit office environment. Occasional evening and weekend work.

Mental/Physical Requirements:
- Lifting—Not to exceed 50 lbs.
- Writing, sitting, bending, visual acuity, reading, field of vision/peripheral
- Standing—spends majority of the shift working on their feet
- Regularly required to use hands to finger, handle, or feel objects, tools, or controls; bend, reach with hands and arms; stoop, kneel, and talk and/or hear.
- Exposure to: noise, chemical vapors, infectious materials
- Combination of sitting, standing, bending, light lifting and walking.
- Requires a full range of body motion including manual and finger dexterity and hand-eye coordination.

- Requires corrected vision and hearing to a normal range.
- Requires the ability to manage stressful situations.
- Occasional stress from varying demands.

Disclaimer: This description is intended to provide only basic guidelines for meeting job requirements. Responsibilities, knowledge, skills, abilities and working conditions may change as needs of the organization evolve.

Job Title: Front Desk/Check-In
Department: Administration
Immediate Supervisor Title: Front Desk Manager
Job Supervisory Responsibilities: None

General Summary:

- Essential Job Responsibilities:
- Greets patients and visitors to the practice
- Registers patients in the practice management system which may mean entering information given verbally or on registration forms
- Collects identification and insurance cards and copies or scans them for the record, may photograph the patient for the record
- May collect co-pays or other monies
- Prints encounter form (also called superbill, routing slip, or fee ticket) with updated information, or updates information on the encounter form
- Has patient sign financial agreement, receipt of privacy policy, benefits assignment, etc.
- May answer phone calls, take messages, and make appointments
- Directs visitors appropriately

Education:

Experience:

Other Requirements:

- Must be available to have a mixed schedule of opening and closing the office and the ability to be flexible with schedule when needed.

Competency Requirements:

Knowledge:

- Knowledge of organizational policies, procedures, and systems.
- Knowledge of office management techniques and practices.
- Knowledge of computer systems, programs, and applications.
- Knowledge of grammar, spelling, and punctuation.
- General knowledge of healthcare terminology preferred.
- Knowledge of purchasing, budgeting, and inventory control.

Skills:

- Ability to communicate in English, both verbally and in writing.
- Additional languages preferred.
- Must possess strong human relations, communication, problem solving, and organizational skills to interact with a variety of customers and personnel, both within and outside the institution.
- Must be able to work independently and in a team environment.
- Requires strong personal computer skills, communication skills, problem solving, continuous improvement and teaming skills.
- Maintains a broad knowledge of clinical, financial, and administrative systems/applications and processes.
- Serves as a resource on department and institutional initiatives; shares knowledge with customers and colleagues.
- Demonstrated verbal and written communication skills.

Abilities:

- Must maintain regular and acceptable attendance; may be required to work weekend, holiday or OT hours.

- Ability to establish and maintain effective working relationships with other employees and the public.
- Ability to work under pressure, communicate and present information.
- Ability to read, interpret, and apply clinic policies and procedures.
- Ability to identify problems, recommend solutions, organize and analyze information.
- Ability to establish priorities and coordinate work activities.
- Exposure to electronic health record preferred.
- Ability to work independently, be goal-directed and have strong organizational skills.
- Effectively multitask without compromising quality.
- Ability to comprehend and excel in both verbal and written communication, including proper telephone etiquette, face-to-face interactions, and electronic communications.
- Ability to communicate with individuals and small groups with credibility and confidence.
- Ability to handle difficult situations, remain calm under stress, manage emotional situations, display empathy and maintain positive communication during a rapidly changing/dynamic environment.
- Turn problems into opportunities by developing innovative and creative solutions.
- Demonstrate a friendly, positive attitude, display energy and drive in performing daily responsibilities.

- Must be flexible as well as easily adapt to a changing work environment which will require ongoing maintenance of job-related skills/activities.
- Must be willing to adjust work schedules in response to department or clinical needs.
- Able to manage and prioritize tasks simultaneously while working directly with patients who may exhibit diverse needs.

Equipment Operated:

- Standard office equipment including computers, fax machines, copiers, printers, telephones, etc.

Work Environment:

- Position is in a well-lit office environment. Occasional evening and weekend work.

Mental/Physical Requirements:

- Involves sitting approximately 90 percent of the day, walking or standing the remainder.
- Combination of sitting, standing, bending, light lifting and walking.
- Requires a full range of body motion including manual and finger dexterity and hand-eye coordination.
- Requires corrected vision and hearing to a normal range.
- Requires the ability to manage stressful situations.
- Occasional stress from varying demands.

Disclaimer: This description is intended to provide only basic guidelines for meeting job requirements. Responsibilities, knowledge, skills, abilities and working conditions may change as needs of the organization evolve.

Job Title: Front desk clerk

Department: Administration
Immediate Supervisor Title: Office Manager
Job Supervisory Responsibilities:

General Summary:

- Essential Job Responsibilities:
- Greets patients and visitors to the practice
- Registers patients in the practice management system which may mean entering information given verbally or on registration forms
- Collects identification and insurance cards and copies or scans them for the record, may photograph the patient for the record
- May collect co-pays or other monies
- Prints encounter form (also called superbill, routing slip, or fee ticket) with updated information, or updates information on the encounter form
- Has patient sign financial agreement, receipt of privacy policy, benefits assignment, etc.
- May answer phone calls, take messages and make appointments
- Directs visitor (drug reps, salespersons, etc.) appropriately

Education:

- High school diploma or GED and one year of customer service experience required, such as administrative, physician's office, appointment scheduler or retail/ service industry. Associate degree and coursework in a healthcare related field is preferred (e.g., Administrative Clinic Assistant, Medical Office, Medical Assistant, Healthcare/Medical Receptionist or comparable).

- Requires computer skills including Windows-based applications and intranet/internet use with the ability to keyboard and navigate through multiple applications.
- Basic Life Support (BLS) may be required in some areas.
- Individuals may also need to complete additional coursework upon hire.
- Individuals that have not completed a Medical Terminology course will be required to successfully complete a Medical Terminology course within six months of employment.

Experience:

- Minimum two years of administrative experience, including one year with a health care organization.
- [Medical specialty] office experience is a plus.

Other Requirements:

- Must be available to have a mixed schedule of opening and closing the office and the ability to be flexible with schedule when needed.

Competency Requirements:

Knowledge:

- Knowledge of and experience with [vendor-specific EHR] is preferred
- Knowledge of proper phone etiquette and phone handling skills
- Knowledge of organizational policies, procedures, and systems.
- Knowledge of office management techniques and practices.
- Knowledge of computer systems, programs, and applications.
- Knowledge of research methods and procedures sufficient to compile data and prepare reports.

- Knowledge of grammar, spelling, and punctuation.
- General knowledge of healthcare terminology preferred.
- Knowledge of purchasing, budgeting, and inventory control.

Skills:

- Skill in taking and transcribing dictation and in the operation of office equipment.
- Requires strong personal computer skills, communication skills, problem solving, continuous improvement and teaming skills.
- Maintains a broad knowledge of this practice's clinical, financial, and administrative systems/applications and processes.
- Serves as a resource on department and institutional initiatives; shares knowledge with customers and colleagues.
- Demonstrated verbal and written communication skills.

Abilities:

- Must maintain regular and acceptable attendance; may be required to work weekend, holiday or OT hours.
- Ability to establish and maintain effective working relationships with other employees and the public.
- Ability to work under pressure, communicate and present information.
- Ability to read, interpret, and apply clinic policies and procedures.
- Ability to identify problems, recommend solutions, organize and analyze information.
- Ability to establish priorities and coordinate work activities.
- Exposure to electronic health record preferred.
- Ability to work independently, be goal-directed and have strong organizational skills.
- Effectively multitask without compromising quality.

- Ability to comprehend and excel in both verbal and written communication, including proper telephone etiquette, face-to-face interactions, and electronic communications.
- Ability to communicate with individuals and small groups with credibility and confidence.
- Ability to handle difficult situations, remain calm under stress, manage emotional situations, display empathy and maintain positive communication during a rapidly changing/dynamic environment.
- Turn problems into opportunities by developing innovative and creative solutions.
- Demonstrate a friendly, positive attitude, display energy and drive in performing daily responsibilities.
- Must be flexible as well as easily adapt to a changing work environment which will require ongoing maintenance of job-related skills/activities.
- Must be willing to adjust work schedules in response to department or clinical needs.
- Able to manage and prioritize tasks simultaneously while working directly with patients who may exhibit diverse needs.

Equipment Operated:

- Standard office equipment including computers, fax machines, copiers, printers, telephones, etc.

Work Environment:

- Position is in a well-lit office environment. Occasional evening and weekend work.

Mental/Physical Requirements:

- Involves sitting approximately 90 percent of the day, walking or standing the remainder.
- Combination of sitting, standing, bending, light lifting and walking.

- Requires a full range of body motion including manual and finger dexterity and hand-eye coordination.
- Requires corrected vision and hearing to a normal range.
- Requires the ability to manage stressful situations.
- Occasional stress from varying demands.

Disclaimer: This description is intended to provide only basic guidelines for meeting job requirements. Responsibilities, knowledge, skills, abilities and working conditions may change as needs of the organization evolve.

Job Title: Medical Records/Health Information Technician

Department: Medical Records, Health Information
Immediate Supervisor Title: Medical Records, Health Information, or Clinical Services Manager
Job Supervisory Responsibilities: None

General Summary:

- An administrative position responsible for assembling patient information into patients' medical charts/records in accurate and complete manner
- Position responsibilities vary by size of medical practice and type of technology used such as electronic medical records versus manual files.

Essential Job Responsibilities:

- Assembles patients' health information including patient symptoms and medical history, exam results, X-ray reports, lab tests, diagnoses, and treatment plans. Checks to ensure all forms are completed, properly identified, and signed and that all necessary information is in the manual and/or computer file in preferred manner such as chronological.
- Enhance patient experiences; optimizing company reputation.
- Ensure compliance with current healthcare regulations, medical laws, federal and state laws, and high ethical standards.
- Communicates as needed with physicians and other health care professionals to clarify diagnoses or to obtain additional information.
- Submits files/documentation to physicians and other clinicians as requested for review, quality assurance checks, and other purposes.

- Provides charts/documents requested for use in legal actions, following patient consent/confidentiality protocols.
- Codes patients' information periodically (as back-up) for insurance purposes. Assigns a code to each diagnosis and procedure (diagnosis-related group [DRG]).
- Uses computer programs if requested to tabulate and analyze data to improve patient care, control costs, respond to surveys, or use in research studies.

Education:

- High school diploma or GED and one year of customer service experience required, such as administrative, physician's office, appointment scheduler or retail/ service industry.
- Associate degree and coursework in a healthcare related field is preferred (e.g., Administrative Clinic Assistant, Medical Office, Medical Assistant, Healthcare/Medical Receptionist or comparable).

Experience:

- [Medical specialty] office experience is a plus.
- Minimum two years of medical records clerk/health information technician experience, preferably in medical practice setting.

Other Requirements:

- Must be available to have a mixed schedule of opening and closing the office and the ability to be flexible with schedule when needed.
- Registered health information technician (RHIT) designation preferred, but not required. Offered by the American Health Information Management Association; designation awarded after successfully completing written exam.

Competency Requirements:

Knowledge:

- Knowledge of and experience with [vendor-specific EHR] is preferred.
- Knowledge of Electronic Health Systems in any case
- Knowledge of Practice Management Systems
- Knowledge of biology, chemistry, health, and computer science.
- Knowledge of medical terminology.
- Knowledge of legal and ethical considerations related to patient information.

Skills:

- Skill in putting information in preferred medical record system, meeting clinic standards.
- Skill in dealing with masses of information in organized manner.
- Skill in using computer and medical records software.

Abilities:

- Must maintain regular and acceptable attendance; may be required to work weekend, holiday or OT hours.
- Ability to establish and maintain effective working relationships with other employees and the public.
- Ability to work under pressure, communicate and present information.
- Ability to read, interpret, and apply clinic policies and procedures.
- Ability to identify problems, recommend solutions, organize and analyze information.
- Ability to establish priorities and coordinate work activities.
- Exposure to electronic health record preferred.
- Ability to work independently, be goal-directed and have strong organizational skills.
- Effectively multitask without compromising quality.

- Ability to comprehend and excel in both verbal and written communication, including proper telephone etiquette, face-to-face interactions, and electronic communications.
- Ability to communicate with individuals and small groups with credibility and confidence.
- Ability to alphabetize and put information (materials, forms, etc.) into chronological order.
- Ability to analyze medical records for completeness and accuracy, paying attention to detail.
- Ability to schedule time and assignments effectively.

Equipment Operated:

- Standard office equipment including computers, fax machines, copiers, printers, telephones, etc.
- Range of medical records equipment and supplies, including computer hardware/ software, manual files, and sorters.

Work Environment:

- Position is in a well-lit office environment. Occasional evening and weekend work.

Mental/Physical Requirements:

- Involves sitting approximately 90 % of the day, walking or standing the remainder.
- Combination of sitting, standing, bending, light lifting and walking.
- Requires a full range of body motion including manual and finger dexterity and hand-eye coordination.
- Requires corrected vision and hearing to a normal range.
- Requires the ability to manage stressful situations.
- Occasional stress from varying demands.

Disclaimer: This description is intended to provide only basic guidelines for meeting job requirements. Responsibilities, knowledge, skills, abilities and working conditions may change as needs of the organization evolve.

Job Title: Financial Analyst

Department: Accounting
Immediate Supervisor Title: Accounting Manager
Job Supervisory Responsibilities: Designated
individuals in the accounting department

General Summary:

- A professional position responsible for assisting in determining financial objectives; analyzing and reporting accounting variances; developing and monitoring accounting reports and control mechanisms.
- Analyzes financial status by collecting, monitoring, and studying data; recommending actions.

Essential Job Responsibilities:

- Determines cost of operations by establishing standard costs; collecting operational data.
- Identifies financial status by comparing and analyzing actual results with plans and forecasts.
- Guides cost analysis process by establishing and enforcing policies and procedures; providing trends and forecasts; explaining processes and techniques; recommending actions.
- Improves financial status by analyzing results; monitoring variances; identifying trends; recommending actions to management.
- Reconciles transactions by comparing and correcting data.
- Maintains database by entering, verifying, and backing up data.
- Recommends actions by analyzing and interpreting data and making comparative analyses; studying proposed changes in methods and materials.

- Increases productivity by developing automated accounting applications; coordinating information requirements.
- Protects operations by keeping financial information confidential.
- Maintains technical knowledge by attending educational workshops; reviewing publications.
- Contributes to team effort by accomplishing related results as needed.

Education:

- Certified Public Accountant certificate.
- Bachelor's degree in accounting or finance.
- Individuals may also need to complete additional coursework upon hire.
- Individuals that have not completed a Medical Terminology course will be required to successfully complete a Medical Terminology course within six months of employment.

Experience:

- Minimum three years of experience in accounting management, including two years in a health care organization.

Other Requirements:

- Must be available to have a mixed schedule of opening and closing the office and the ability to be flexible with schedule when needed.
- MGMA certification.
- CPA required.

Competency Requirements

Knowledge:

- Knowledge of and experience with [vendor-specific EHR] is preferred.
- Knowledge of Electronic Health Systems in any case
- Knowledge of Practice Management Systems
- Knowledge of proper phone etiquette and phone handling skills.
- Knowledge of organizational policies, procedures, and systems.
- Knowledge of office management techniques and practices.
- Knowledge of computer systems, programs, and applications.
- Knowledge of grammar, spelling, and punctuation.
- General knowledge of healthcare terminology preferred.
- Knowledge of purchasing, budgeting, and inventory control.
- Knowledge of advanced financial accounting, analysis, and reporting to design, modify, and manage an accounting system.
- Knowledge of automated accounting systems and governmental regulations.
- Knowledge of reimbursement procedures to compile and allocate cost information to specific accounts.

Skills:

- Skill in taking and transcribing dictation and in the operation of office equipment.
- This position requires strong working knowledge of managed care plans, insurance carriers, referrals and precertification procedures.
- Ability to communicate in English, both verbally and in writing.
- Additional languages preferred.
- CPT and ICD-10 coding abilities preferred.

- Must possess strong human relations, communication, problem solving, and organizational skills to interact with a variety of customers and personnel, both within and outside the institution.
- Must be able to work independently and in a team environment.
- Requires strong personal computer skills, communication skills, problem solving, continuous improvement and teaming skills.
- Maintains a broad knowledge of clinical, financial, and administrative systems/applications and processes.
- Serves as a resource on department and institutional initiatives; shares knowledge with customers and colleagues.
- Demonstrated verbal and written communication skills.
- Skill in budgeting, preparing financial reports, and computer applications.
- Skill in exercising initiative, judgment, discretion, and decision-making to achieve organizational objectives.
- Skill in identifying and resolving accounting problems.

Abilities:
- Must maintain regular and acceptable attendance; may be required to work weekend, holiday or OT hours.
- Ability to establish and maintain effective working relationships with other employees and the public.
- Ability to work under pressure, communicate and present information.
- Ability to read, interpret, and apply clinic policies and procedures.
- Ability to identify problems, recommend solutions, organize and analyze information.
- Ability to establish priorities and coordinate work activities.
- Exposure to electronic health record preferred.
- Ability to work independently, be goal-directed and have strong organizational skills.

- Effectively multitask without compromising quality.
- Ability to comprehend and excel in both verbal and written communication, including proper telephone etiquette, face-to-face interactions, and electronic communications.
- Ability to communicate with individuals and small groups with credibility and confidence.
- Ability to handle difficult situations, remain calm under stress, manage emotional situations, display empathy and maintain positive communication during a rapidly changing/dynamic environment.
- Turn problems into opportunities by developing innovative and creative solutions.
- Demonstrate a friendly, positive attitude, display energy and drive in performing daily responsibilities.
- Must be flexible as well as easily adapt to a changing work environment which will require ongoing maintenance of job-related skills/activities.
- Must be willing to adjust work schedules in response to department or clinical needs.
- Able to manage and prioritize tasks simultaneously while working directly with patients who may exhibit diverse needs. Ability to delegate responsibility and authority to staff.
- Ability to work creatively with management and department staff to achieve objectives.
- Ability to communicate effectively with all levels of management regarding financial policies.

Equipment Operated:
- Standard office equipment including computers, fax machines, copiers, printers, telephones, etc.

Work Environment:
- Position is in a well-lit office environment. Occasional evening and weekend work.

Mental/Physical Requirements:

- Involves sitting approximately 90 percent of the day, walking or standing the remainder.
- Combination of sitting, standing, bending, light lifting and walking.
- Requires a full range of body motion including manual and finger dexterity and hand-eye coordination.
- Requires corrected vision and hearing to a normal range.
- Requires the ability to manage stressful situations.
- Occasional stress from varying demands.

Disclaimer: This description is intended to provide only basic guidelines for meeting job requirements. Responsibilities, knowledge, skills, abilities and working conditions may change as needs of the organization evolve.

Job Title: Billing and Follow-up
Department: Finance
Immediate Supervisor Title: Comptroller
Job Supervisory Responsibilities: Medical Coder

General Summary:

- A non-clinical position responsible for collection of delinquent patient accounts.
- Corrects claims that are rejected from the claim's scrubber, clearinghouse or payer.
- Files secondary and tertiary claims as needed, electronically or via paper.
- Posts receipts from insurance companies and patients and edits any electronic remittance advice; may post from lockbox account on the web.
- May prepare deposits and/or make deposits.
- Generates patient statements.
- May check eligibility on patients with appointments and call patients whose insurance is not active .
- Calls patients who have not made payments in response to statements.
- May turn patients over to third-party collectors.
- Takes phone calls from payers or patients about billing issues and resolves issues.

Essential Job Responsibilities:

- Identifies delinquent accounts, aging period, and payment sources. Processes delinquent unpaid accounts by contacting patients and third-party reimbursors.
- Reviews accounts, credit reports, and other information sources such as credit bureaus via computer.
- Ensure compliance with current healthcare regulations, medical laws, federal and state laws, and high ethical standards.

- Performs various collection actions including contacting patients by phone and resubmitting claims to third-party reimbursors.
- Evaluates patient financial status and establishes budget payment plans.
- Follows and reports status of delinquent accounts.
- Reviews accounts for possible assignment; makes recommendations to credit manager and prepares information for collection agency.
- Assigns uncollectible accounts to collection agency or attorney via clinic credit and collection policy.
- Contacts lawyers involved in third-party litigation.

Education:

- High school diploma or equivalent. Some college preferred.

Experience:

- Minimum two years of medical collections experience.

Competency Requirements:

Knowledge:

- Knowledge of medical billing/collection practices.
- Knowledge of basic medical coding and third-party operating procedures and practices.
- Knowledge of legal and regulatory government provisions.

Skills:

- Skill in establishing and maintaining effective internal and external working relationships.

Abilities:

- Ability to enter accurately data and examine insurance documents.

- Ability to deal courteously with patients, staff, and others.
- Ability to communicate effectively and clearly.

Equipment Operated:

- Standard office equipment including computers, fax machines, copiers, printers, telephones, etc.

Work Environment:

- Position is in a well-lit office environment. Occasional evening and weekend work.

Mental/Physical Requirements:

- Involves sitting approximately 90 percent of the day, walking or standing the remainder.
- Combination of sitting, standing, bending, light lifting and walking.
- Requires a full range of body motion including manual and finger dexterity and hand-eye coordination.
- Requires corrected vision and hearing to a normal range.
- Requires the ability to manage stressful situations.
- Occasional stress from varying demands.

Job Title: Billing Specialist

Department: Billing
Immediate Supervisor Title: : Office Supervisor
Job Supervisory Responsibilities: None

General Summary:

- The Billing Specialist immediately communicates any identified problems that may affect cash flow to the account payable representative.
- In addition to the day-to-day billing activities, The Billing Specialist assesses the billing cycles and anticipates problem areas for early intervention.

Essential Job Responsibilities:

- Maintain a file of billing requirements for major insurers.
- Maintains computer billing master tables.
- Post insurance and patient payments.
- Enter heart station billing.
- Collect and enter cardiac catheterization and interventional billing.
- Collect and enter all inpatient billing charges.
- Submit claims on a timely basis.
- Timely follow-up on unpaid claims.
- Review reports to evaluate claims status.
- Investigate and resolve patient/insurance company inquiries concerning services, billing, or fees/charges.
- Notify patient and insurance company, as well as other appropriate personnel, of findings, adjustments, and recommendations.
- Contact insurer if not paid within 30 days.
- Locate and notify patient/insurance company of delinquent accounts by mail or telephone to solicit payment.

- Perform billing duties utilizing specific knowledge of medical terminology and hospital and office procedures.
- E-mail pertinent department correspondence to all staff in order to facilitate on-going communications and efficient department operations.
- Maintain appropriate levels of the supplies necessary to complete assigned responsibilities.
- Maintain dignity and respect for all patients, family members, staff, visitors and clinic personnel.
- Maintain attendance and punctuality to ensure the department is operated in an efficient and cost-effective manner.
- Utilize spare time in work-related activities, which contribute to the clinic's needs.
- Coordinate efforts to effectively work with others in a manner that is productive.
- Be depended on to modify work schedule as required.
- Interact with fellow employees in a way that promotes a harmonious and cooperative working environment.
- Participate and present at the "Lunch and Learn" sessions.

Education:

- Associate degree and coursework in an Accounting or Healthcare related field is preferred (e.g., Administrative Clinic Assistant, Medical Office, Medical Assistant, Healthcare/Medical Receptionist or comparable).
- Basic Life Support (BLS) may be required in some areas.
- Individuals may also need to complete additional coursework upon hire.
- Individuals that have not completed a Medical Terminology course will be required to successfully complete a Medical Terminology course within six months of employment.

Experience:

- Minimum two years of administrative experience, including one year with a health care organization.
- [Medical specialty] office experience is a plus.

Other Requirements:

- Must be available to have a mixed schedule of opening and closing the office and the ability to be flexible with schedule when needed.

Competency Requirements:

Knowledge:

- Knowledge of policies and procedures to manage operations and ensure effective patient care.
- Knowledge of the principles and practices of health care administration, fiscal management, and government regulations and reimbursements.
- Knowledge of Electronic Health Systems.
- Knowledge of Practice Management Systems.
- Knowledge of proper phone etiquette and phone handling skills.
- Knowledge of organizational policies, procedures, and systems.
- Knowledge of office management techniques and practices.
- Knowledge of computer systems, programs, and applications.
- Knowledge of research methods and procedures sufficient to compile data and prepare reports.
- Knowledge of grammar, spelling, and punctuation.
- General knowledge of healthcare terminology preferred.
- Knowledge of purchasing, budgeting, and inventory control.

Skills:

- This position requires strong working knowledge of managed care plans, insurance carriers, referrals and precertification procedures.
- Skill in exercising a high degree of initiative, judgment, and discretion.
- Skill in analyzing situations accurately and taking effective action.
- Skill in establishing and maintaining effective working relationships.
- Skill in organizing work, delegating and achieving goals and objectives.
- Skill in exercising judgment and discretion in developing, interpreting, and implementing departmental policies and procedures.
- Ability to communicate in English, both verbally and in writing.
- Additional languages preferred.
- Must possess strong human relations, communication, problem solving, and organizational skills to interact with a variety of customers and personnel, both within and outside the institution.
- Must be able to work independently and in a team environment.
- Requires strong personal computer skills, communication skills, problem solving, continuous improvement and teaming skills.
- Maintains a broad knowledge of clinical, financial, and administrative systems/applications and processes.
- Serves as a resource on department and institutional initiatives; shares knowledge with customers and colleagues.
- Demonstrated verbal and written communication skills.

Abilities:

- Must maintain regular and acceptable attendance; may be required to work weekend, holiday or OT hours.
- Ability to establish and maintain effective working relationships with other employees and the public.
- Ability to work under pressure, communicate and present information.
- Ability to read, interpret, and apply clinic policies and procedures.
- Ability to identify problems, recommend solutions, organize and analyze information.
- Ability to establish priorities and coordinate work activities.
- Exposure to electronic health record preferred.
- Ability to work independently, be goal-directed and have strong organizational skills.
- Effectively multitask without compromising quality.
- Ability to comprehend and excel in both verbal and written communication, including proper telephone etiquette, face-to-face interactions, and electronic communications.
- Ability to communicate with individuals and small groups with credibility and confidence.
- Ability to handle difficult situations, remain calm under stress, manage emotional situations, display empathy and maintain positive communication during a rapidly changing/dynamic environment.
- Turn problems into opportunities by developing innovative and creative solutions.
- Demonstrate a friendly, positive attitude, display energy and drive in performing daily responsibilities.
- Must be flexible as well as easily adapt to a changing work environment which will require ongoing maintenance of job-related skills/activities.
- Must be willing to adjust work schedules in response to department or clinical needs.

Equipment Operated:

- Standard office equipment including computers, fax machines, copiers, printers, telephones, etc.

Work Environment:

- Position is in a well-lit office environment.
- Occasional evening and weekend work.

Mental/Physical Requirements:

- Involves sitting approximately 90 percent of the day, walking or standing the remainder.
- Combination of sitting, standing, bending, light lifting and walking.
- Requires a full range of body motion including manual and finger dexterity and hand-eye coordination.
- Lifting up to 20 pounds.
- Requires corrected vision and hearing to a normal range.
- Requires the ability to manage stressful situations.
- Occasional stress from varying demands.

Disclaimer: This description is intended to provide only basic guidelines for meeting job requirements. Responsibilities, knowledge, skills, abilities and working conditions may change as needs of the organization evolve.

Job Title: Medical Coder

Department: Administration
Immediate Supervisor Title: Office Manager, Billing Manager, Comptroller
Job Supervisory Responsibilities: None

General Summary:

- Medical Coders work for healthcare facilities where they convert patients' information to standardized codes, which are used on documentation for healthcare insurance claims and for databases.
- Medical Coders assist practitioners to receive reimbursement from healthcare insurance companies, Medicaid and Medicare.
- The Medical Coder will assign required CPT, HCPCS, ICD-10-CM, and ASA codes.
- Assign APC or DRG codes.

Essential Job Responsibilities:

- Reviews notes from inpatient or outpatient encounters and codes them according to the documentation
- May post charges for services rendered.
- Audits chart documentation for quality purposes to ensure that provider coding and documentation is synchronous.
- Make judicious decisions on which codes to assign in each instance, and function to a high level of accuracy.
- Introduces changes in procedure (HCPCS) and diagnosis (ICD-10) codes and educates staff on the use of new codes.
- Ensures encounter forms and practice management software is updated appropriately with new and deleted codes.
- May be delegated the role of practice Compliance Officer.

- Liaising with physicians and other parties to clarify information.
- Examining documents for missing information.
- Assigning CPT, HCPCS, ICD-10-CM, and ASA codes.
- Assigning APC and DRG codes.
- Ensuring documents are grammatically correct and free from typing errors.
- Performing chart audits.
- Advising and training physicians and staff on medical coding.
- Informing supervisor of issues with equipment and computer program.
- Ensuring compliance with medical coding policies and guidelines.

Education:

- Certification in Medical coding for Medicare, Medicaid and major medical plans.
- High school diploma or GED and one year of customer service experience required, such as administrative, physician's office, appointment scheduler or retail/service industry.
- Requires computer skills, including Windows-based applications and intranet/internet use with the ability to keyboard and navigate through multiple applications.
- Individuals that have not completed a Medical Terminology course will be required to successfully complete a Medical Terminology course within six months of employment.

Additional qualifications:

- Associate degree and coursework in a healthcare related field is preferred (e.g., Administrative Clinic Assistant, Medical Office, Medical Assistant, Healthcare/Medical Receptionist or comparable).
- Exposure to electronic health record preferred.

- Ability to work independently, be goal-directed and have strong organizational skills.
- Effectively multitask without compromising quality.
- Ability to comprehend and excel in both verbal and written communication, including proper telephone etiquette, face-to-face interactions, and electronic communications.
- Ability to communicate with individuals and small groups with credibility and confidence.
- Ability to handle difficult situations, remain calm under stress, manage emotional situations, display empathy and maintain positive communication during a rapidly changing/dynamic environment.
- Turn problems into opportunities by developing innovative and creative solutions.
- Demonstrate a friendly, positive attitude, display energy and drive in performing daily responsibilities.
- Must be flexible as well as easily adapt to a changing work environment which will require ongoing maintenance of job-related skills/activities.
- Must be willing to adjust work schedules in response to department or clinical needs.
- Able to manage and prioritize tasks simultaneously while working directly with patients who may exhibit diverse needs.
- Basic Life Support (BLS) may be required in some areas.
- Individuals may also need to complete additional coursework upon hire.

Experience:

- Minimum two years of administrative experience, including one year with a health care organization.
- [Medical specialty] office experience is a plus.

Other Requirements:

- Must be available to have a mixed schedule of opening and closing the office and the ability to be flexible with schedule when needed.

Competency Requirements:

Knowledge:

- Knowledge of and experience with [vendor-specific EHR] is preferred
- Knowledge of proper phone etiquette and phone handling skills
- Knowledge of organizational policies, procedures, and systems.
- Knowledge of office management techniques and practices.
- Knowledge of computer systems, programs, and applications.
- Knowledge of research methods and procedures sufficient to compile data and prepare reports.
- Knowledge of grammar, spelling, and punctuation.
- General knowledge of healthcare terminology preferred.
- Knowledge of purchasing, budgeting, and inventory control.

Skills:

- Skill in taking and transcribing dictation and in the operation of office equipment.
- Requires strong personal computer skills, communication skills, problem solving, continuous improvement and teaming skills.
- Maintains a broad knowledge of practice's clinical, financial, and administrative systems/applications and processes.
- Demonstrated verbal and written communication skills.

Abilities:

- Must maintain regular and acceptable attendance; may be required to work weekend, holiday or OT hours.
- Ability to establish and maintain effective working relationships with other employees and the public.
- Ability to work under pressure, communicate and present information.
- Ability to read, interpret, and apply clinic policies and procedures.
- Ability to identify problems, recommend solutions, organize and analyze information.
- Ability to establish priorities and coordinate work activities.

Equipment Operated:

- Standard office equipment including computers, fax machines, copiers, printers, telephones, etc.

Work Environment:

- Position is in a well-lit office environment. Occasional evening and weekend work.

Mental/Physical Requirements:

- Involves sitting approximately 90 percent of the day, walking or standing the remainder.
- Combination of sitting, standing, bending, light lifting and walking.
- Requires a full range of body motion including manual and finger dexterity and hand-eye coordination.
- Requires corrected vision and hearing to a normal range.
- Requires the ability to manage stressful situations.
- Occasional stress from varying demands.

Disclaimer: This description is intended to provide only basic guidelines for meeting job requirements. Responsibilities, knowledge, skills, abilities and working conditions may change as needs of the organization evolve.

Job Title: Coding Analyst-Denial Management

Department: Administration
Immediate Supervisor Title: Office Manager, Practice Manager, Comptroller
Job Supervisory Responsibilities: Medical Coder

General Summary:

- The Denial Management Coding Analyst supports the denial management team by reviewing claims for coding accuracy and root causes for coding-related denials, as well as proposing process improvements to mitigate future denials. Working closely alongside the Physician Advisor, the Denial Management Coding Analyst liaises between the denial management team, coding operations, and providers, resolving queries for missing documentation and promoting departmental awareness of coding best practices. This position will serve as a resource for Denial Management Coders needing assistance resolving complex denials and may provide direction to those staff regarding priorities and productivity goals.

- A Denial Management Coding Analyst will also research and resolve coding denials via [vendor-specific EHR] work queues, and process charge corrections based on medical record reviews, contracts, regulations, in accordance with this practice's policies. This position is also required to interpret and review physician-professional documentation in validating procedural, supplies, drugs and diagnosis coding for the professional claims. A Denial Management Coding Analyst is also responsible for reviewing hospital inpatient or hospital outpatient documentation in validating claim ICD-10-CM diagnosis codes, ICD-10-PCS codes, and CPT-4 procedural codes for UB-04 Outpatient or Inpatient claims. This position will defend the claim and seek payment from the payer by facilitating resolution of the denial through resubmission of supporting documentation, including discussion(s) with the payer or via the payer's website.

Essential Job Responsibilities:

Education:

- Registered Health Information Administrator (RHIA), Registered Health Information Technician (RHIT), or coding credential of a Certified Coding Specialist (CCS) or Certified Professional Coder (CPC) required.
- Associate's degree in a health care related area required; Bachelor's degree is preferred.

Experience:

- Minimum of 4 years of physician/professional or hospital outpatient coding experience or minimum of 6 years of relevant hospital inpatient coding experience including DRG assignment.

Other Requirements:

- Must be available to have a mixed schedule of opening and closing the office and the ability to be flexible with schedule when needed.

Competency Requirements:

Knowledge:

- Knowledge of professional/physician coding rules for inpatient, hospital outpatient, clinic, and/ or emergency settings. Experience with National Correct Coding Initiative (NCCI) edits, National Coverage Determinations (NCD), Local Coverage Determinations (LCD), and outpatient coding guidelines for official coding and reporting.

- In-depth knowledge of medical terminology, disease processes, patient health record content and the medical record coding process.
- Knowledge of principles, methods, and techniques related to compliant healthcare billing/collections.
- Familiarity with provider-based billing (PBB) and critical access hospital (CAH) coding and billing requirements is a plus.
- Demonstrated ability to partner with physicians and provide feedback on medical documentation best practices.
- Knowledge of grammar, spelling, and punctuation.
- General knowledge of healthcare terminology.
- Knowledge of and experience with [vendor-specific EHR] is preferred.

Skills:

- Skill in taking and transcribing dictation and in the operation of office equipment.
- Requires strong personal computer skills, communication skills, problem solving, continuous improvement and teaming skills.
- Maintains a broad knowledge of this practice's clinical, financial, and administrative systems/applications and processes.
- Serves as a resource on department and institutional initiatives; shares knowledge with customers and colleagues.
- Demonstrated verbal and written communication skills.

Abilities:

- Must maintain regular and acceptable attendance; may be required to work weekend, holiday or OT hours.
- Ability to establish and maintain effective working relationships with other employees and the public.
- Ability to work under pressure, communicate and present information.

- Ability to read, interpret, and apply clinic policies and procedures.
- Ability to identify problems, recommend solutions, organize and analyze information.
- Ability to establish priorities and coordinate work activities.
- Ability to work independently, be goal-directed and have strong organizational skills.
- Effectively multitask without compromising quality.
- Ability to comprehend and excel in both verbal and written communication, including proper telephone etiquette, face-to-face interactions, and electronic communications.
- Ability to communicate with individuals and small groups with credibility and confidence.
- Ability to handle difficult situations, remain calm under stress, manage emotional situations, display empathy and maintain positive communication during a rapidly changing/dynamic environment.
- Turn problems into opportunities by developing innovative and creative solutions.
- Demonstrate a friendly, positive attitude, display energy and drive in performing daily responsibilities.
- Must be flexible as well as easily adapt to a changing work environment which will require ongoing maintenance of job-related skills/activities.

Equipment Operated:

- Standard office equipment including computers, fax machines, copiers, printers, telephones, etc.

Work Environment:

- Position is in a well-lit office environment. Occasional evening and weekend work.

Mental/Physical Requirements:

- Involves sitting approximately 90 percent of the day, walking or standing the remainder.
- Combination of sitting, standing, bending, light lifting and walking.
- Requires a full range of body motion including manual and finger dexterity and hand-eye coordination.
- Requires corrected vision and hearing to a normal range.
- Requires the ability to manage stressful situations.
- Occasional stress from varying demands.

Disclaimer: This description is intended to provide only basic guidelines for meeting job requirements. Responsibilities, knowledge, skills, abilities and working conditions may change as needs of the organization evolve.

Job Title: Medical Claims Specialist/Examiner
Department: Billing
Immediate Supervisor Title: : Office Supervisor
Job Supervisory Responsibilities: None

General Summary:

- Serves medical insurance customers by determining insurance coverage; examining and resolving medical claims; documenting actions; maintaining quality customer services; ensuring legal compliance.

Essential Job Responsibilities:

- Determines covered medical insurance losses by studying provisions of policy or certificate.
- Establishes proof of loss by studying medical documentation; assembling additional information as required from outside sources, including claimant, physician, employer, hospital, and other insurance companies; initiating or conducting investigation of questionable claims.
- Documents medical claims actions by completing forms, reports, logs, and records.
- Resolves medical claims by approving or denying documentation; calculating benefit due; initiating payment or composing denial letter.
- Ensures legal compliance by following company policies, procedures, guidelines, as well as state and federal insurance regulations.
- Maintains quality customer services by following customer service practices; responding to customer inquiries.
- Provides legal support by assembling documentation for settlement action.
- Protects operations by keeping claims information confidential.

- Prepares reports by collecting, analyzing, and summarizing information.
- Updates job knowledge by participating in educational opportunities; reading professional publications; maintaining personal networks; participating in professional organizations.
- Accomplishes organization goals by accepting ownership for accomplishing new and different requests; exploring opportunities to add value to job accomplishments.

Education:

- Associate degree and coursework in an Accounting or Healthcare related field is preferred (e.g., Administrative Clinic Assistant, Medical Office, Medical Assistant, Healthcare/Medical Receptionist or comparable).
- Basic Life Support (BLS) may be required in some areas.
- Individuals may also need to complete additional coursework upon hire.
- Individuals that have not completed a Medical Terminology course will be required to successfully complete a Medical Terminology course within six months of employment.

Experience:

- Minimum two years of administrative experience, including one year with a health care organization.

Other Requirements:

- Must be available to have a mixed schedule of opening and closing the office and the ability to be flexible with schedule when needed.

Competency Requirements:

Knowledge:

- Knowledge of policies and procedures to manage operations and ensure effective patient care.
- Knowledge of the principles and practices of health care administration, fiscal management, and government regulations and reimbursements.
- Knowledge of Electronic Health Systems.
- Knowledge of Practice Management Systems.
- Knowledge of proper phone etiquette and phone handling skills.
- Knowledge of organizational policies, procedures, and systems.
- Knowledge of office management techniques and practices.
- Knowledge of computer systems, programs, and applications.
- Knowledge of research methods and procedures sufficient to compile data and prepare reports.
- Knowledge of grammar, spelling, and punctuation.
- General knowledge of healthcare terminology preferred.
- Knowledge of purchasing, budgeting, and inventory control.

Skills:

- This position requires strong working knowledge of managed care plans, insurance carriers, referrals and precertification procedures.
- Skill in exercising a high degree of initiative, judgment, and discretion.
- Skill in analyzing situations accurately and taking effective action.
- Skill in establishing and maintaining effective working relationships.
- Skill in organizing work, delegating and achieving goals and objectives.

- Skill in exercising judgment and discretion in developing, interpreting, and implementing departmental policies and procedures.
- Ability to communicate in English, both verbally and in writing.
- Additional languages preferred.
- Must possess strong human relations, communication, problem solving, and organizational skills to interact with a variety of customers and personnel, both within and outside the institution.
- Must be able to work independently and in a team environment.
- Requires strong personal computer skills, communication skills, problem solving, continuous improvement and teaming skills.
- Maintains a broad knowledge of clinical, financial, and administrative systems/applications and processes.
- Serves as a resource on department and institutional initiatives; shares knowledge with customers and colleagues.
- Demonstrated verbal and written communication skills.

Abilities:

- Must maintain regular and acceptable attendance; may be required to work weekend, holiday or OT hours.
- Ability to establish and maintain effective working relationships with other employees and the public.
- Ability to work under pressure, communicate and present information.
- Ability to read, interpret, and apply clinic policies and procedures.
- Ability to identify problems, recommend solutions, organize and analyze information.
- Ability to establish priorities and coordinate work activities.
- Exposure to electronic health record preferred.

- Ability to work independently, be goal-directed and have strong organizational skills.
- Effectively multitask without compromising quality.
- Ability to comprehend and excel in both verbal and written communication, including proper telephone etiquette, face-to-face interactions, and electronic communications.
- Ability to communicate with individuals and small groups with credibility and confidence.
- Ability to handle difficult situations, remain calm under stress, manage emotional situations, display empathy and maintain positive communication during a rapidly changing/dynamic environment.
- Turn problems into opportunities by developing innovative and creative solutions.
- Demonstrate a friendly, positive attitude, display energy and drive in performing daily responsibilities.
- Must be flexible as well as easily adapt to a changing work environment which will require ongoing maintenance of job-related skills/activities.
- Must be willing to adjust work schedules in response to department or clinical needs.

Equipment Operated:

- Standard office equipment including computers, fax machines, copiers, printers, telephones, etc.

Work Environment:

- Position is in a well-lit office environment.
- Occasional evening and weekend work.

Mental/Physical Requirements:

- Lifting—Not to exceed 50 lbs.
- Writing, sitting, bending, visual acuity, reading, field of vision/peripheral

- Standing—spends majority of the shift working on their feet
- Regularly required to use hands to finger, handle, or feel objects, tools, or controls; bend, reach with hands and arms; stoop, kneel, and talk and/or hear.
- Exposure to: noise, chemical vapors, infectious materials
- Combination of sitting, standing, bending, light lifting and walking.
- Requires a full range of body motion including manual and finger dexterity and hand-eye coordination.
- Requires corrected vision and hearing to a normal range.
- Requires the ability to manage stressful situations.
- Occasional stress from varying demands.

Disclaimer: This description is intended to provide only basic guidelines for meeting job requirements. Responsibilities, knowledge, skills, abilities and working conditions may change as needs of the organization evolve.

Job Title: Patient Account Representative
Department: Administration
Immediate Supervisor Title: Office Manager
Job Supervisory Responsibilities: None

General Summary:

- Institutional Insurance and reimbursement expert for one or more of the following business lines: outpatient pharmacy, durable medical equipment, skilled nursing facility, home health agency or continuing care retirement center.
- Performs all aspects of the billing and collection processes for the individual business lines across the enterprise.
- These processes include service pre-certification, insurance coverage review and personal responsibility determination, communications with patients, claim submissions, denial review, rebilling, appeals, and accounts receivable management.
- Utilizes skills in problem solving, customer service, and communications (verbal and written) in interactions with patients and internal customers to resolve a variety of account, billing and payment issues for patients, physicians, nurses, pharmacists, technicians and social workers. Interprets, applies and communicates
- Clinic policies regarding financial aspects of patient care to assure optimal reimbursement for both the patient and the Clinic.

Essential Job Responsibilities:

- Enhance patient experiences; optimizing company reputation.
- Ensure compliance with current healthcare regulations, medical laws, federal and state laws, and high ethical standards.

Education:

- Associate degree in finance, business or healthcare related majors and one year experience in medical, pharmacy or durable medical equipment billing and collection activities.
- Or high school diploma/GED with at least 3 years' experience in medical, pharmacy or durable medical equipment billing and collection activities.

Experience:

- One year experience in medical, pharmacy or durable medical equipment billing and collection activities.

Other Requirements:

- Must be available to have a mixed schedule of opening and closing the office and the ability to be flexible with schedule when needed.

Competency Requirements:

Knowledge:

- Knowledge of and experience with [vendor-specific EHR] is preferred.
- Knowledge of Electronic Health Systems in any case
- Knowledge of Practice Management Systems
- Knowledge of proper phone etiquette and phone handling skills.
- Knowledge of organizational policies, procedures, and systems.
- Knowledge of office management techniques and practices.
- Knowledge of computer systems, programs, and applications.
- Knowledge of research methods and procedures sufficient to compile data and prepare reports.
- Knowledge of grammar, spelling, and punctuation.

- General knowledge of healthcare terminology preferred.
- Knowledge of purchasing, budgeting, and inventory control.

Skills:

- Skill in taking and transcribing dictation and in the operation of office equipment.
- This position requires strong working knowledge of managed care plans, insurance carriers, referrals and precertification procedures.
- Ability to communicate in English, both verbally and in writing.
- Additional languages preferred.
- Associate degree coding abilities preferred.
- Must possess strong human relations, communication, problem solving, and organizational skills to interact with a variety of customers and personnel, both within and outside the institution.
- Must be able to work independently and in a team environment.
- Requires strong personal computer skills, communication skills, problem solving, continuous improvement and teaming skills.
- Maintains a broad knowledge of clinical, financial, and administrative systems/applications and processes.
- Serves as a resource on department and institutional initiatives; shares knowledge with customers and colleagues.
- Demonstrated verbal and written communication skills.

Abilities:

- Must maintain regular and acceptable attendance; may be required to work weekend, holiday or OT hours.
- Ability to establish and maintain effective working relationships with other employees and the public.
- Ability to work under pressure, communicate and present information.

- Ability to read, interpret, and apply clinic policies and procedures.
- Ability to identify problems, recommend solutions, organize and analyze information.
- Ability to establish priorities and coordinate work activities.
- Exposure to electronic health record preferred.
- Ability to work independently, be goal-directed and have strong organizational skills.
- Effectively multitask without compromising quality.
- Ability to comprehend and excel in both verbal and written communication, including proper telephone etiquette, face-to-face interactions, and electronic communications.
- Ability to communicate with individuals and small groups with credibility and confidence.
- Ability to handle difficult situations, remain calm under stress, manage emotional situations, display empathy and maintain positive communication during a rapidly changing/dynamic environment.
- Turn problems into opportunities by developing innovative and creative solutions.
- Demonstrate a friendly, positive attitude, display energy and drive in performing daily responsibilities.
- Must be flexible as well as easily adapt to a changing work environment which will require ongoing maintenance of job-related skills/activities.
- Must be willing to adjust work schedules in response to department or clinical needs.
- Able to manage and prioritize tasks simultaneously while working directly with patients who may exhibit diverse needs.

Equipment Operated:
- Standard office equipment including computers, fax machines, copiers, printers, telephones, etc.

Work Environment:

- Position is in a well-lit office environment. Occasional evening and weekend work.

Mental/Physical Requirements:

- Involves sitting approximately 90 percent of the day, walking or standing the remainder.
- Combination of sitting, standing, bending, light lifting and walking.
- Requires a full range of body motion including manual and finger dexterity and hand-eye coordination.
- Requires corrected vision and hearing to a normal range.
- Requires the ability to manage stressful situations.
- Occasional stress from varying demands.

Disclaimer: This description is intended to provide only basic guidelines for meeting job requirements. Responsibilities, knowledge, skills, abilities and working conditions may change as needs of the organization evolve.

Job Title: Business Analyst

Department: Accounting
Immediate Supervisor Title: Accounting Manager
Job Supervisory Responsibilities: None

General Summary:

- Business Analyst will use transactional data and statistical methods to provide insight into business Competency and suggest area and methods of improving operations.
- The Business Analyst is accountable for implementing and overseeing the analytical approaches and methodologies for the department and ensures that project/department milestones/goals are met and are in compliance with approved budgets.
- The Business Analyst is responsible for presenting insight and recommendations to management for decision making and strategic planning.

Essential Job Responsibilities:

- Support business initiatives through data analysis, identification of implementation barriers and user acceptance testing of various systems
- Manage site quotas and file size limits on SharePoint— maintain and optimize the enterprise SharePoint search engine
- Deliver detailed requirements.
- Serve as the liaison between internal and external customers/users and development team to gather, analyze, interpret, clarify, and develop business requirements on the assigned projects; ensure that projects are meeting the requirements during each phase
- Develop and maintain a variety of documents including project charter, ROI analysis, business

requirements, specifications, roadmaps, and other business documentation as required by the department

- Partner with software development team and ensure business requirements are provided to them and understood as an input for their technical documentation and collaborate with them throughout project life cycle
- Diagnose problems and identify opportunities for process redesign and improvement
- Produce monthly metrics reporting at the end of each month
- Prioritize operational reporting requests on behalf of the operations

Education:

- Advanced degree in Business Administration, Accounting, Finance or related field
- Individuals that have not completed a Medical Terminology course will be required to successfully complete a Medical Terminology course within six months of employment.

Experience:

- Minimum three years of administrative experience, including one year with a health care organization.

Other Requirements:

- Must be available to have a mixed schedule of opening and closing the office and the ability to be flexible with schedule when needed.
- MGMA certification.

Competency Requirements:

Knowledge:

- Knowledge of organizational policies, procedures, and systems.
- Knowledge of office management techniques and practices.
- Knowledge of computer systems, programs, and applications.
- Knowledge of grammar, spelling, and punctuation.
- General knowledge of healthcare terminology preferred.
- Knowledge of purchasing, budgeting, and inventory control.

Skills:

- Ability to communicate in English, both verbally and in writing.
- Additional languages preferred.
- Must possess strong human relations, communication, problem solving, and organizational skills to interact with a variety of customers and personnel, both within and outside the institution.
- Must be able to work independently and in a team environment.
- Requires strong personal computer skills, communication skills, problem solving, continuous improvement and teaming skills.
- Maintains a broad knowledge of clinical, financial, and administrative systems/applications and processes.
- Serves as a resource on department and institutional initiatives; shares knowledge with customers and colleagues.
- Demonstrated verbal and written communication skills.

Abilities:

- Must maintain regular and acceptable attendance; may be required to work weekend, holiday or OT hours.

- Ability to establish and maintain effective working relationships with other employees and the public.
- Ability to work under pressure, communicate and present information.
- Ability to read, interpret, and apply clinic policies and procedures.
- Ability to identify problems, recommend solutions, organize and analyze information.
- Ability to establish priorities and coordinate work activities.
- Exposure to electronic health record preferred.
- Ability to work independently, be goal-directed and have strong organizational skills.
- Effectively multitask without compromising quality.
- Ability to comprehend and excel in both verbal and written communication, including proper telephone etiquette, face-to-face interactions, and electronic communications.
- Ability to communicate with individuals and small groups with credibility and confidence.
- Ability to handle difficult situations, remain calm under stress, manage emotional situations, display empathy and maintain positive communication during a rapidly changing/dynamic environment.
- Turn problems into opportunities by developing innovative and creative solutions.
- Demonstrate a friendly, positive attitude, display energy and drive in performing daily responsibilities.
- Must be flexible as well as easily adapt to a changing work environment which will require ongoing maintenance of job-related skills/activities.
- Must be willing to adjust work schedules in response to department or clinical needs.
- Able to manage and prioritize tasks simultaneously while working directly with patients who may exhibit diverse needs.

Equipment Operated:

- Standard office equipment including computers, fax machines, copiers, printers, telephones, etc.

Work Environment:

- Position is in a well-lit office environment. Occasional evening and weekend work.

Mental/Physical Requirements:

- Involves sitting approximately 90 percent of the day, walking or standing the remainder.
- Combination of sitting, standing, bending, light lifting and walking.
- Requires a full range of body motion including manual and finger dexterity and hand-eye coordination.
- Requires corrected vision and hearing to a normal range.
- Requires the ability to manage stressful situations.
- Occasional stress from varying demands.

Disclaimer: This description is intended to provide only basic guidelines for meeting job requirements. Responsibilities, knowledge, skills, abilities and working conditions may change as needs of the organization evolve.

Job Title: Director of Operations

Department: Administration
Immediate Supervisor Title: Front Desk Manager
Job Supervisory Responsibilities: Front Desk/Check-In

General Summary:

- Responsible for the smooth operation of the practice, coordinating administration, clinical and facilities functions.

Essential Job Responsibilities:

- Maintain and continue to develop an organizational culture at both the company office as well as urgent care center locations to achieve ongoing excellence and effective growth with the highest integrity.
- Lead the successful development of existing urgent care centers.
- Lead the timely opening of new urgent care centers.
- Coordinate with chief medical officer and medical directors to ensure delivery of quality patient care and achieve patient satisfaction.
- Lead senior practice administrator in the day-to-day management of center operations.
- Lead marketing department in various community and outreach activities.
- Lead marketing department in the development and implementation of processes at each center to deliver upon existing and newly contract services.
- Serve as liaison to medical billing and coding team.
- Ensure compliance at each center as to federal, state and local law in clinical as well as general business operations.
- Overall, ensure synergies among people, process, and strategies to drive execution of business and healthcare objectives.

Education:

- Advanced degree in Business Administration, Accounting, Finance or related field
- Individuals that have not completed a Medical Terminology course will be required to successfully complete a Medical Terminology course within six months of employment.

Experience:

- Minimum ten years of administrative experience, including one year with a health care organization.

Other Requirements:

- Must be available to have a mixed schedule of opening and closing the office and the ability to be flexible with schedule when needed.
- MGMA certification.

Competency Requirements:

Knowledge:

- Knowledge of organizational policies, procedures, and systems.
- Knowledge of office management techniques and practices.
- Knowledge of computer systems, programs, and applications.
- Knowledge of grammar, spelling, and punctuation.
- General knowledge of healthcare terminology preferred.
- Knowledge of purchasing, budgeting, and inventory control.

Skills:

- Ability to communicate in English, both verbally and in writing.
- Additional languages preferred.

- Must possess strong human relations, communication, problem solving, and organizational skills to interact with a variety of customers and personnel, both within and outside the institution.
- Must be able to work independently and in a team environment.
- Requires strong personal computer skills, communication skills, problem solving, continuous improvement and teaming skills.
- Maintains a broad knowledge of clinical, financial, and administrative systems/applications and processes.
- Serves as a resource on department and institutional initiatives; shares knowledge with customers and colleagues.
- Demonstrated verbal and written communication skills.

Abilities:
- Must maintain regular and acceptable attendance; may be required to work weekend, holiday or OT hours.
- Ability to establish and maintain effective working relationships with other employees and the public.
- Ability to work under pressure, communicate and present information.
- Ability to read, interpret, and apply clinic policies and procedures.
- Ability to identify problems, recommend solutions, organize and analyze information.
- Ability to establish priorities and coordinate work activities.
- Exposure to electronic health record preferred.
- Ability to work independently, be goal-directed and have strong organizational skills.
- Effectively multitask without compromising quality.
- Ability to comprehend and excel in both verbal and written communication, including proper telephone etiquette, face-to-face interactions, and electronic communications.

- Ability to communicate with individuals and small groups with credibility and confidence.
- Ability to handle difficult situations, remain calm under stress, manage emotional situations, display empathy and maintain positive communication during a rapidly changing/dynamic environment.
- Turn problems into opportunities by developing innovative and creative solutions.
- Demonstrate a friendly, positive attitude, display energy and drive in performing daily responsibilities.
- Must be flexible as well as easily adapt to a changing work environment which will require ongoing maintenance of job-related skills/activities.
- Must be willing to adjust work schedules in response to department or clinical needs.
- Able to manage and prioritize tasks simultaneously while working directly with patients who may exhibit diverse needs.

Equipment Operated:

- Standard office equipment including computers, fax machines, copiers, printers, telephones, etc.

Work Environment:

- Position is in a well-lit office environment. Occasional evening and weekend work.

Mental/Physical Requirements:

- Involves sitting approximately 90 percent of the day, walking or standing the remainder.
- Combination of sitting, standing, bending, light lifting and walking.
- Requires a full range of body motion including manual and finger dexterity and hand-eye coordination.
- Requires corrected vision and hearing to a normal range.

- Requires the ability to manage stressful situations.
- Occasional stress from varying demands.

Disclaimer: This description is intended to provide only basic guidelines for meeting job requirements. Responsibilities, knowledge, skills, abilities and working conditions may change as needs of the organization evolve.

Job Title: Medical Office Manager
Department: Administration
Immediate Supervisor Title: Practice Administrator
Job Supervisory Responsibilities: Front office staff

General Summary:

- Under the general direction of the Practice Administrator, the Medical Office Manager is responsible for the overall supervision of the office personnel and functions as a full working member of the clinic floating to areas in the office that require assistance.
- The Medical Office Manager is also responsible for managing employee work flow with administrative functions of the Clinic including but not limited to business operations, clinical operations, and patient billing/accounting responsibilities.
- The Medical Office Manager prepares work schedules and manages staff time and attendance weekly for payroll.
- Responsible for ordering and performing inventory on office supplies for all clinics.
- Keeps the physician(s) informed of both progress and potential problems.
- Works with all staff for the direction and evaluation of patient care delivery.
- Monitors activities continually with the billing collection company, collection agencies, insurance companies, patients and physicians; recommends corrective action as appropriate.
- Trains and assists staff as appropriate.
- Facilitates patient visits and supports the health care provider by anticipating and responding to patient needs and requests of the health care team.

Essential Job Responsibilities:

- Enhance patient experiences; optimizing company reputation.
- Ensure compliance with current healthcare regulations, medical laws, federal and state laws, and high ethical standards.

Education:

- Associate degree and one year of customer service experience required, such as administrative, physician's office, appointment scheduler or retail/service industry.
- Graduate of a medical office specialist program highly preferred.
- Requires computer skills including Windows-based applications and intranet/internet use with the ability to keyboard and navigate through multiple applications.
- Basic Life Support (BLS) may be required in some areas.
- Individuals may also need to complete additional coursework upon hire.
- Individuals that have not completed a Medical Terminology course will be required to successfully complete a Medical Terminology course within six months of employment.

Experience:

- Minimum two years of administrative experience, including one year with a health care organization.
- [Medical specialty] office experience is a plus.
- Three Years previous Practice Management experience highly preferred.

Other Requirements:

- Must be available to have a mixed schedule of opening and closing the office and the ability to be flexible with schedule when needed.

Competency Requirements:

Knowledge:

- Knowledge of and experience with [vendor-specific EHR] is preferred.
- Knowledge of proper phone etiquette and phone handling skills.
- Knowledge of organizational policies, procedures, and systems.
- Knowledge of office management techniques and practices.
- Knowledge of computer systems, programs, and applications.
- Knowledge of research methods and procedures sufficient to compile data and prepare reports.
- Knowledge of grammar, spelling, and punctuation.
- General knowledge of healthcare terminology preferred.
- Knowledge of purchasing, budgeting, and inventory control.

Skills:

- Skill in taking and transcribing dictation and in the operation of office equipment.
- Ability to communicate in English, both verbally and in writing.
- Additional languages preferred.
- CPT and ICD-10 coding abilities preferred.
- Requires strong personal computer skills, communication skills, problem solving, continuous improvement and teaming skills.
- Maintains a broad knowledge of clinical, financial, and administrative systems/applications and processes.
- Serves as a resource on department and institutional initiatives; shares knowledge with customers and colleagues.
- Demonstrated verbal and written communication skills.

Abilities:

- Must maintain regular and acceptable attendance; may be required to work weekend, holiday or OT hours.
- Ability to establish and maintain effective working relationships with other employees and the public.
- Ability to work under pressure, communicate and present information.
- Ability to read, interpret, and apply clinic policies and procedures.
- Ability to identify problems, recommend solutions, organize and analyze information.
- Ability to establish priorities and coordinate work activities.
- Exposure to electronic health record preferred.
- Ability to work independently, be goal-directed and have strong organizational skills.
- Effectively multitask without compromising quality.
- Ability to comprehend and excel in both verbal and written communication, including proper telephone etiquette, face-to-face interactions, and electronic communications.
- Ability to communicate with individuals and small groups with credibility and confidence.
- Ability to handle difficult situations, remain calm under stress, manage emotional situations, display empathy and maintain positive communication during a rapidly changing/dynamic environment.
- Turn problems into opportunities by developing innovative and creative solutions.
- Demonstrate a friendly, positive attitude, display energy and drive in performing daily responsibilities.
- Must be flexible as well as easily adapt to a changing work environment which will require ongoing maintenance of job-related skills/activities.
- Must be willing to adjust work schedules in response to department or clinical needs.

- Able to manage and prioritize tasks simultaneously while working directly with patients who may exhibit diverse needs.

Equipment Operated:

- Standard office equipment including computers, fax machines, copiers, printers, telephones, etc.

Work Environment:

- Position is in a well-lit office environment. Occasional evening and weekend work.

Mental/Physical Requirements:

- Lifting—Not to exceed 50 lbs.
- Writing, sitting, bending, visual acuity, reading, field of vision/peripheral
- Standing—spends majority of the shift working on their feet
- Regularly required to use hands to finger, handle, or feel objects, tools, or controls; bend, reach with hands and arms; stoop, kneel, and talk and/or hear.
- Exposure to: noise, chemical vapors, infectious materials
- Combination of sitting, standing, bending, light lifting and walking.
- Requires a full range of body motion including manual and finger dexterity and hand-eye coordination.
- Requires corrected vision and hearing to a normal range.
- Requires the ability to manage stressful situations.
- Occasional stress from varying demands.

Disclaimer: This description is intended to provide only basic guidelines for meeting job requirements. Responsibilities, knowledge, skills, abilities and working conditions may change as needs of the organization evolve.

Job Title: Billing Coordinator

Department: Administration
Immediate Supervisor Title: Office Supervisor
Job Supervisory Responsibilities: Billing/Coding staff

General Summary:

- Immediately communicates any identified problems that may affect cash flow to the accounts payable representative.
- Assesses the billing cycles and anticipates problem areas for early intervention.

Essential Job Responsibilities:

- Maintain a file of billing requirements for major insurers.
- Maintains computer billing master tables.
- Post insurance and patient payments.
- Enter heart station billing.
- Collect and enter cardiac catheterization and interventional billing.
- Collect and enter all inpatient billing charges.

Under the direct supervision of the office supervisor:

- Submit claims on a timely basis.
- Timely follow-up on unpaid claims.
- Review reports to evaluate claims status.
- Investigate and resolve patient/insurance company inquiries concerning services, billing, or fees/charges. Notify patient/insurance company and appropriate personnel of findings, adjustments, and recommendations.
- Contact insurer if not paid within 30 days.
- Locate and notify patient/insurance company of delinquent accounts by mail or telephone to solicit payment.

- Perform billing duties utilizing specific knowledge of medical terminology and hospital and office procedures
- E-mail pertinent department correspondence to all staff in order to facilitate on-going communications and efficient department operations.
- Maintain appropriate levels of the supplies necessary to complete assigned responsibilities.
- Maintain dignity and respect for all patients, family members, staff, visitors and clinic personnel.
- Maintain attendance and punctuality to ensure the department is operated in an efficient and cost-effective manner.
- Utilize spare time in work-related activities, which contribute to the clinic's needs.
- Coordinate efforts to effectively work with others in a manner that is productive.
- Be depended on to modify work schedule as required.
- Interact with fellow employees in a way that promotes a harmonious and cooperative working environment.
- Participate and present at the "Lunch and Learn" sessions.

Education:

- Associate degree and coursework in a healthcare related field is preferred (e.g., Administrative Clinic Assistant, Medical Office, Medical Assistant, Healthcare/Medical Receptionist or comparable).
- Bachelor's degree in Business Administration or health-related field
- Basic Life Support (BLS) may be required in some areas.
- Individuals may also need to complete additional coursework upon hire.
- Individuals that have not completed a Medical Terminology course will be required to successfully complete a Medical Terminology course within six months of employment.

Experience:

- Minimum two years of administrative experience, including one year with a health care organization.
- [Medical specialty] office experience is a plus.

Other Requirements:

- Must be available to have a mixed schedule of opening and closing the office and the ability to be flexible with schedule when needed.
- MGMA certification.

Competency Requirements:

Knowledge:

- Knowledge of and experience with [vendor-specific EHR] is preferred.
- Knowledge of Electronic Health Systems in any case
- Knowledge of Practice Management Systems
- Knowledge of proper phone etiquette and phone handling skills.
- Knowledge of organizational policies, procedures, and systems.
- Knowledge of office management techniques and practices.
- Knowledge of computer systems, programs, and applications.
- Knowledge of research methods and procedures sufficient to compile data and prepare reports.
- Knowledge of grammar, spelling, and punctuation.
- General knowledge of healthcare terminology preferred.
- Knowledge of purchasing, budgeting, and inventory control.

Skills:

- Skill in taking and transcribing dictation and in the operation of office equipment.

- This position requires strong working knowledge of managed care plans, insurance carriers, referrals and precertification procedures.
- Ability to communicate in English, both verbally and in writing.
- Additional languages preferred.
- CPT and ICD-10 coding abilities preferred.
- Must possess strong human relations, communication, problem solving, and organizational skills to interact with a variety of customers and personnel, both within and outside the institution.
- Must be able to work independently and in a team environment.
- Requires strong personal computer skills, communication skills, problem solving, continuous improvement and teaming skills.
- Maintains a broad knowledge of clinical, financial, and administrative systems/applications and processes.
- Serves as a resource on department and institutional initiatives; shares knowledge with customers and colleagues.
- Demonstrated verbal and written communication skills.

Abilities:

- Must maintain regular and acceptable attendance; may be required to work weekend, holiday or OT hours.
- Ability to establish and maintain effective working relationships with other employees and the public.
- Ability to work under pressure, communicate and present information.
- Ability to read, interpret, and apply clinic policies and procedures.
- Ability to identify problems, recommend solutions, organize and analyze information.
- Ability to establish priorities and coordinate work activities.
- Exposure to electronic health record preferred.

- Ability to work independently, be goal-directed and have strong organizational skills.
- Effectively multitask without compromising quality.
- Ability to comprehend and excel in both verbal and written communication, including proper telephone etiquette, face-to-face interactions, and electronic communications.
- Ability to communicate with individuals and small groups with credibility and confidence.
- Ability to handle difficult situations, remain calm under stress, manage emotional situations, display empathy and maintain positive communication during a rapidly changing/dynamic environment.
- Turn problems into opportunities by developing innovative and creative solutions.
- Demonstrate a friendly, positive attitude, display energy and drive in performing daily responsibilities.
- Must be flexible as well as easily adapt to a changing work environment which will require ongoing maintenance of job-related skills/activities.
- Must be willing to adjust work schedules in response to department or clinical needs.
- Able to manage and prioritize tasks simultaneously while working directly with patients who may exhibit diverse needs.

Equipment Operated:

- Standard office equipment including computers, fax machines, copiers, printers, telephones, etc.

Work Environment:

- Position is in a well-lit office environment. Occasional evening and weekend work.

Mental/Physical Requirements:

- Involves sitting approximately 90 percent of the day, walking or standing the remainder.
- Combination of sitting, standing, bending, light lifting and walking.
- Requires a full range of body motion including manual and finger dexterity and hand-eye coordination.
- Requires corrected vision and hearing to a normal range.
- Requires the ability to manage stressful situations.
- Occasional stress from varying demands.

Disclaimer: This description is intended to provide only basic guidelines for meeting job requirements. Responsibilities, knowledge, skills, abilities and working conditions may change as needs of the organization evolve.

Job Title: Billing Manager

Department: Administration
Immediate Supervisor Title: Office Supervisor
Job Supervisory Responsibilities: Billing/Coding staff

General Summary:

- Immediately communicates any identified problems that may affect cash flow to the accounts payable representative.
- Assesses the billing cycles and anticipates problem areas for early intervention.

Essential Job Responsibilities:

- Supervising Billing/Coding department, verifying the following is completed correctly:
- Maintain a file of billing requirements for major insurers.
- Maintains computer billing master tables.
- Post insurance and patient payments.
- Enter heart station billing.
- Collect and enter cardiac catheterization and interventional billing.
- Collect and enter all inpatient billing charges.
- Under the direct supervision of the office supervisor:
- Submit claims on a timely basis.
- Timely follow-up on unpaid claims.
- Review reports to evaluate claims status.
- Investigate and resolve patient/insurance company inquiries concerning services, billing, or fees/charges. Notify patient/insurance company and appropriate personnel of findings, adjustments, and recommendations.
- Contact insurer if not paid within 30 days.

- Locate and notify patient/insurance company of delinquent accounts by mail or telephone to solicit payment.
- Perform billing duties utilizing specific knowledge of medical terminology and hospital and office procedures
- E-mail pertinent department correspondence to all staff in order to facilitate on-going communications and efficient department operations.
- Maintain appropriate levels of the supplies necessary to complete assigned responsibilities.
- Maintain dignity and respect for all patients, family members, staff, visitors and clinic personnel.
- Maintain attendance and punctuality to ensure the department is operated in an efficient and cost-effective manner.
- Utilize spare time in work-related activities, which contribute to the clinic's needs.
- Coordinate efforts to effectively work with others in a manner that is productive.
- Be depended on to modify work schedule as required.
- Interact with fellow employees in a way that promotes a harmonious and cooperative working environment.
- Participate and present at the "Lunch and Learn" sessions.

Education:

- Associate degree and coursework in a healthcare related field is preferred (e.g., Administrative Clinic Assistant, Medical Office, Medical Assistant, Healthcare/Medical Receptionist or comparable).
- Bachelor's degree in Business Administration or health-related field
- Basic Life Support (BLS) may be required in some areas.
- Individuals may also need to complete additional coursework upon hire.

- Individuals that have not completed a Medical Terminology course will be required to successfully complete a Medical Terminology course within six months of employment.

Experience:

- Minimum two years of administrative experience, including one year with a health care organization.
- [Medical specialty] office experience is a plus.

Other Requirements:

- Must be available to have a mixed schedule of opening and closing the office and the ability to be flexible with schedule when needed.

Competency Requirements:

Knowledge:

- Knowledge of and experience with [vendor-specific EHR] is preferred.
- Knowledge of Electronic Health Systems in any case
- Knowledge of Practice Management Systems
- Knowledge of proper phone etiquette and phone handling skills.
- Knowledge of organizational policies, procedures, and systems.
- Knowledge of office management techniques and practices.
- Knowledge of computer systems, programs, and applications.
- Knowledge of research methods and procedures sufficient to compile data and prepare reports.
- Knowledge of grammar, spelling, and punctuation.
- General knowledge of healthcare terminology preferred.
- Knowledge of purchasing, budgeting, and inventory control.

Skills:

- Skill in taking and transcribing dictation and in the operation of office equipment.
- This position requires strong working knowledge of managed care plans, insurance carriers, referrals and precertification procedures.
- Ability to communicate in English, both verbally and in writing.
- Additional languages preferred.
- CPT and ICD-10 coding abilities preferred.
- Must possess strong human relations, communication, problem solving, and organizational skills to interact with a variety of customers and personnel, both within and outside the institution.
- Must be able to work independently and in a team environment.
- Requires strong personal computer skills, communication skills, problem solving, continuous improvement and teaming skills.
- Maintains a broad knowledge of clinical, financial, and administrative systems/applications and processes.
- Serves as a resource on department and institutional initiatives; shares knowledge with customers and colleagues.
- Demonstrated verbal and written communication skills.

Abilities:

- Must maintain regular and acceptable attendance; may be required to work weekend, holiday or OT hours.
- Ability to establish and maintain effective working relationships with other employees and the public.
- Ability to work under pressure, communicate and present information.
- Ability to read, interpret, and apply clinic policies and procedures.

- Ability to identify problems, recommend solutions, organize and analyze information.
- Ability to establish priorities and coordinate work activities.
- Exposure to electronic health record preferred.
- Ability to work independently, be goal-directed and have strong organizational skills.
- Effectively multitask without compromising quality.
- Ability to comprehend and excel in both verbal and written communication, including proper telephone etiquette, face-to-face interactions, and electronic communications.
- Ability to communicate with individuals and small groups with credibility and confidence.
- Ability to handle difficult situations, remain calm under stress, manage emotional situations, display empathy and maintain positive communication during a rapidly changing/dynamic environment.
- Turn problems into opportunities by developing innovative and creative solutions.
- Demonstrate a friendly, positive attitude, display energy and drive in performing daily responsibilities.
- Must be flexible as well as easily adapt to a changing work environment which will require ongoing maintenance of job-related skills/activities.
- Must be willing to adjust work schedules in response to department or clinical needs.
- Able to manage and prioritize tasks simultaneously while working directly with patients who may exhibit diverse needs.

Equipment Operated:

- Standard office equipment including computers, fax machines, copiers, printers, telephones, etc.

Work Environment:

- Position is in a well-lit office environment. Occasional evening and weekend work.

Mental/Physical Requirements:

- Involves sitting approximately 90 percent of the day, walking or standing the remainder.
- Combination of sitting, standing, bending, light lifting and walking.
- Requires a full range of body motion including manual and finger dexterity and hand-eye coordination.
- Requires corrected vision and hearing to a normal range.
- Requires the ability to manage stressful situations.
- Occasional stress from varying demands.

Disclaimer: This description is intended to provide only basic guidelines for meeting job requirements. Responsibilities, knowledge, skills, abilities and working conditions may change as needs of the organization evolve.

Job Title: Physician Office Manager
Department: Administration
Immediate Supervisor Title: Practice Administrator
Job Supervisory Responsibilities: Clinical staff

General Summary:

- Under the general direction of the Practice Administrator, the Physician Office Manager is responsible for the overall supervision of the Clinical administration personnel and functions as a full working member of the clinic floating to areas in the clinic that require assistance.
- The Physician Office Manager is also responsible for managing employee work flow with administrative functions of the Clinic including but not limited to business operations, clinical operations, and patient billing/accounting responsibilities.
- The Physician Office Manager prepares work schedules and manages staff time and attendance weekly for payroll.
- Responsible for ordering and performing inventory on office supplies for all clinics.
- Keeps the physician(s) informed of both progress and potential problems.
- Works with all staff for the direction and evaluation of patient care delivery.
- Monitors activities continually with the billing collection company, collection agencies, insurance companies, patients and physicians; recommends corrective action as appropriate.
- Trains and assists staff as appropriate.
- Facilitates patient visits and supports the health care provider by anticipating and responding to patient needs and requests of the health care team.

Essential Job Responsibilities:

- Enhance patient experiences; optimizing company reputation.
- Ensure compliance with current healthcare regulations, medical laws, federal and state laws, and high ethical standards.

Education:

- Associate degree and one year of customer service experience required, such as administrative, physician's office, appointment scheduler or retail/service industry.
- Graduate of a medical office specialist program highly preferred.
- Requires computer skills including Windows-based applications and intranet/internet use with the ability to keyboard and navigate through multiple applications.
- Basic Life Support (BLS) may be required in some areas.
- Individuals may also need to complete additional coursework upon hire.
- Individuals that have not completed a Medical Terminology course will be required to successfully complete a Medical Terminology course within six months of employment.

Experience:

- Minimum two years of administrative experience, including one year with a health care organization.
- [Medical specialty] office experience is a plus.
- Three Years previous Practice Management experience highly preferred.

Other Requirements:

- Must be available to have a mixed schedule of opening and closing the office and the ability to be flexible with schedule when needed.

Competency Requirements:

Knowledge:

- Knowledge of and experience with [vendor-specific EHR] is preferred.
- Knowledge of proper phone etiquette and phone handling skills.
- Knowledge of organizational policies, procedures, and systems.
- Knowledge of office management techniques and practices.
- Knowledge of computer systems, programs, and applications.
- Knowledge of research methods and procedures sufficient to compile data and prepare reports.
- Knowledge of grammar, spelling, and punctuation.
- General knowledge of healthcare terminology preferred.
- Knowledge of purchasing, budgeting, and inventory control.

Skills:

- Skill in taking and transcribing dictation and in the operation of office equipment.
- Ability to communicate in English, both verbally and in writing.
- Additional languages preferred.
- CPT and ICD-10 coding abilities preferred.
- Requires strong personal computer skills, communication skills, problem solving, continuous improvement and teaming skills.
- Maintains a broad knowledge of clinical, financial, and administrative systems/applications and processes.
- Serves as a resource on department and institutional initiatives; shares knowledge with customers and colleagues.
- Demonstrated verbal and written communication skills.

Abilities:

- Must maintain regular and acceptable attendance; may be required to work weekend, holiday or OT hours.
- Ability to establish and maintain effective working relationships with other employees and the public.
- Ability to work under pressure, communicate and present information.
- Ability to read, interpret, and apply clinic policies and procedures.
- Ability to identify problems, recommend solutions, organize and analyze information.
- Ability to establish priorities and coordinate work activities.
- Exposure to electronic health record preferred.
- Ability to work independently, be goal-directed and have strong organizational skills.
- Effectively multitask without compromising quality.
- Ability to comprehend and excel in both verbal and written communication, including proper telephone etiquette, face-to-face interactions, and electronic communications.
- Ability to communicate with individuals and small groups with credibility and confidence.
- Ability to handle difficult situations, remain calm under stress, manage emotional situations, display empathy and maintain positive communication during a rapidly changing/dynamic environment.
- Turn problems into opportunities by developing innovative and creative solutions.
- Demonstrate a friendly, positive attitude, display energy and drive in performing daily responsibilities.
- Must be flexible as well as easily adapt to a changing work environment which will require ongoing maintenance of job-related skills/activities.
- Must be willing to adjust work schedules in response to department or clinical needs.

- Able to manage and prioritize tasks simultaneously while working directly with patients who may exhibit diverse needs.

Equipment Operated:

- Standard office equipment including computers, fax machines, copiers, printers, telephones, etc.

Work Environment:

- Position is in a well-lit office environment. Occasional evening and weekend work.

Mental/Physical Requirements:

- Lifting—Not to exceed 50 lbs.
- Writing, sitting, bending, visual acuity, reading, field of vision/peripheral
- Standing—spends majority of the shift working on their feet
- Regularly required to use hands to finger, handle, or feel objects, tools, or controls; bend, reach with hands and arms; stoop, kneel, and talk and/or hear.
- Exposure to: noise, chemical vapors, infectious materials
- Combination of sitting, standing, bending, light lifting and walking.
- Requires a full range of body motion including manual and finger dexterity and hand-eye coordination.
- Requires corrected vision and hearing to a normal range.
- Requires the ability to manage stressful situations.
- Occasional stress from varying demands.

Disclaimer: This description is intended to provide only basic guidelines for meeting job requirements. Responsibilities, knowledge, skills, abilities and working conditions may change as needs of the organization evolve.

Job Title: Certified Coding Specialist
Department: Administration
Immediate Supervisor Title: Business Office Manager
Job Supervisory Responsibilities: Business office staff

General Summary:

- Under the direction of the Clinical Operations Supervisor, performs various duties to accurately interpret and bill physician charges for physician services. Entering into the Billing System appropriate CPT and ICD-10 codes bills charges.

Essential Job Responsibilities:

- Performs initial charge review to determine appropriate ICD-10 and CPT codes to be used to report physician services to third party payers.
- Interprets progress notes, operative reports, discharge summaries, and charge documents to determine services provided and accurately assign CPT and ICD-10 coding to these services.
- Enters appropriate data into the [vendor-specific] Billing System by selecting the appropriate codes, diagnosis, modifiers, and times of start and stop of the case, Anesthesiologist, CRNA, and surgeon information to complete the charge process.
- Contacts physicians through management regarding procedures and other services billed to ensure proper coding.
- Responsible for reviewing patient logs and other report of clinical activity to ensure billing is captured for all patients.
- Monitors and follows up to ensure all services that can be billed are captured and coded for billing.
- Responsible for ensuring the batch processes for all coded charges.

- Utilizes batch-logging systems to comply with internal audit standards.
- Reviews all physician documentation to ensure compliance with third party and regulatory guidelines.
- Works in conjunction with the Reimbursement staff to answer all inquiries regarding coding and billing for [vendor-specific] physicians' services.
- Works in coordination with other members of the Physicians' Billing Office as necessary.
- Meets and exceeds short and long term goals as established for the department.
- Performs duties and job functions in accordance with the policies and procedures established for the department.
- Reports to work, meetings and professional obligations on time.
- Participates in administrative staff meetings and attends other meetings and seminars.
- Assists in evaluation of reports, decisions, and results of department in relation to established goals.
- Recommends new approaches, policies, and procedures to influence continuous improvements in department's efficiency and services performed.
- Serves as a member of the Clinical Operations Department. Performs duties necessary to ensure the team's projects/goals are completed.
- Takes ownership of special projects, researches data and follows through with detailed action plans.
- Actively participates in problem identification and resolution and coordinates resolutions between appropriate parties.
- Adheres to Corporate, Department and HR policies and procedures.

Other Requirements:

- Must be available to have a mixed schedule of opening and closing the office and the ability to be flexible with schedule when needed.
- Employee is required to have visual and auditory acuity necessary for communications with other employees and/or customers to meet business needs of [vendor-specific].
- Employee must be able to see written documentation and be able to speak and hear for communication with employees/customers.
- Ability to use a wide array of office equipment including, but not limited to a PC, copier, fax, multi-line telephone, etc.
- Employee is exposed to general indoor working conditions and may on occasion require light lifting or no greater than 20 pounds and some offsite travel.

Education:

- High school diploma or GED and one year of customer service experience required, such as administrative, physician's office, appointment scheduler or retail/ service industry.
- Associate degree and coursework in a healthcare related field is preferred (e.g., Administrative Clinic Assistant, Medical Office, Medical Assistant, Healthcare/Medical Receptionist or comparable).
- Certified Professional Coder with a minimum of two years' experience with CPT and ICD-10 coding of physician services preferred.

Experience:

- Minimum two years of administrative experience, including one year with a health care organization.

Competency Requirements:

Knowledge:

- Knowledge of and experience with [vendor-specific EHR] is preferred.
- Knowledge of Electronic Health Systems in any case
- Knowledge of Practice Management Systems
- Knowledge of proper phone etiquette and phone handling skills.
- Knowledge of organizational policies, procedures, and systems.
- Knowledge of office management techniques and practices.
- Knowledge of computer systems, programs, and applications.
- Knowledge of research methods and procedures sufficient to compile data and prepare reports.
- Knowledge of grammar, spelling, and punctuation.
- General knowledge of healthcare terminology preferred.
- Knowledge of purchasing, budgeting, and inventory control.

Skills:

- Skill in taking and transcribing dictation and in the operation of office equipment.
- This position requires strong working knowledge of managed care plans, insurance carriers, referrals and precertification procedures.
- Ability to communicate in English, both verbally and in writing.
- Additional languages preferred.
- CPT and ICD-10 coding abilities preferred.
- Must possess strong human relations, communication, problem solving, and organizational skills to interact with a variety of customers and personnel, both within and outside the institution.

- Must be able to work independently and in a team environment.
- Requires strong personal computer skills, communication skills, problem solving, continuous improvement and teaming skills.
- Maintains a broad knowledge of clinical, financial, and administrative systems/applications and processes.
- Serves as a resource on department and institutional initiatives; shares knowledge with customers and colleagues.
- Demonstrated verbal and written communication skills.

Abilities:

- Must maintain regular and acceptable attendance; may be required to work weekend, holiday or OT hours.
- Ability to establish and maintain effective working relationships with other employees and the public.
- Ability to work under pressure, communicate and present information.
- Ability to read, interpret, and apply clinic policies and procedures.
- Ability to identify problems, recommend solutions, organize and analyze information.
- Ability to establish priorities and coordinate work activities.
- Exposure to electronic health record preferred.
- Ability to work independently, be goal-directed and have strong organizational skills.
- Effectively multitask without compromising quality.
- Ability to comprehend and excel in both verbal and written communication, including proper telephone etiquette, face-to-face interactions, and electronic communications.
- Ability to communicate with individuals and small groups with credibility and confidence.
- Ability to handle difficult situations, remain calm under stress, manage emotional situations, display empathy

and maintain positive communication during a rapidly changing/dynamic environment.

- Turn problems into opportunities by developing innovative and creative solutions.
- Demonstrate a friendly, positive attitude, display energy and drive in performing daily responsibilities.
- Must be flexible as well as easily adapt to a changing work environment which will require ongoing maintenance of job-related skills/activities.
- Must be willing to adjust work schedules in response to department or clinical needs.
- Able to manage and prioritize tasks simultaneously while working directly with patients who may exhibit diverse needs.

Equipment Operated:

- Standard office equipment including computers, fax machines, copiers, printers, telephones, etc.

Work Environment:

- Position is in a well-lit office environment. Occasional evening and weekend work.

Mental/Physical Requirements:

- Involves sitting approximately 90 percent of the day, walking or standing the remainder.
- Combination of sitting, standing, bending, light lifting and walking.
- Requires a full range of body motion including manual and finger dexterity and hand-eye coordination.
- Requires corrected vision and hearing to a normal range.
- Requires the ability to manage stressful situations.
- Occasional stress from varying demands.

Disclaimer: This description is intended to provide only basic guidelines for meeting job requirements. Responsibilities, knowledge, skills, abilities and working conditions may change as needs of the organization evolve.

Job Title: Appointment Scheduler

Department: Administration
Immediate Supervisor Title: Practice Administrator
Job Supervisory Responsibilities: None

General Summary:

- A position responsible for making appointments for patients following medical practice procedures.

Essential Job Responsibilities:

- Schedules appointments for patients either by phone when they call in or in person after an office visit.
- If medical practice offers after-hours/one-day appointments, schedules these appointments following urgent/emergency protocols as in the case of a sick child, which may mean scheduling the patient with a physician or nurse practitioner other than their primary physician.
- Monitors online appointment request systems and makes sure requests are handled properly.
- Uses manual/computerized system to match physician/clinician availability with patient's preferences in terms of date and time.
- Maintains scheduling system so records are accurate and complete and can be used to analyze patient/staffing patterns. Provides daily schedules to physicians/clinicians or medical assistants prior to each day's visits. Copies also made available to the receptionist/registration clerk and others as needed.
- Ensures that updates (e.g., cancellations or additions) are input daily into master schedule.
- Communicates as needed with physicians/clinicians and other staff about any patient concerns/issues related to scheduling.

- Consults with appointment manager about any system problems.
- Uses customer service principles and techniques to deal with patients calmly and pleasantly.

Education:

- High school diploma or GED and one year of customer service experience required, such as administrative, physician's office, appointment scheduler or retail/service industry.
- Basic Life Support (BLS) may be required in some areas.
- Individuals may also need to complete additional coursework upon hire.
- Individuals that have not completed a Medical Terminology course will be required to successfully complete a Medical Terminology course within six months of employment.

Experience:

- Minimum two years of administrative experience, including one year with a health care organization.
- [Medical specialty] office experience is a plus.

Other Requirements:

- Must be available to have a mixed schedule of opening and closing the office and the ability to be flexible with schedule when needed.

Competency Requirements:

Knowledge:

- Knowledge of and experience with [vendor-specific EHR] is preferred.
- Knowledge of Electronic Health Systems in any case
- Knowledge of Practice Management Systems

- Knowledge of proper phone etiquette and phone handling skills.
- Knowledge of organizational policies, procedures, and systems.
- Knowledge of office management techniques and practices.
- Knowledge of computer systems, programs, and applications.
- Knowledge of research methods and procedures sufficient to compile data and prepare reports.
- Knowledge of grammar, spelling, and punctuation.
- General knowledge of healthcare terminology preferred.
- Knowledge of purchasing, budgeting, and inventory control.

Skills:

- Skill in taking and transcribing dictation and in the operation of office equipment.
- This position requires strong working knowledge of managed care plans, insurance carriers, referrals and precertification procedures.
- Ability to communicate in English, both verbally and in writing.
- Additional languages preferred.
- CPT and ICD-10 coding abilities preferred.
- Must possess strong human relations, communication, problem solving, and organizational skills to interact with a variety of customers and personnel, both within and outside the institution.
- Must be able to work independently and in a team environment.
- Requires strong personal computer skills, communication skills, problem solving, continuous improvement and teaming skills.
- Maintains a broad knowledge of clinical, financial, and administrative systems/applications and processes.

- Serves as a resource on department and institutional initiatives; shares knowledge with customers and colleagues.
- Demonstrated verbal and written communication skills.

Abilities:

- Must maintain regular and acceptable attendance; may be required to work weekend, holiday or OT hours.
- Ability to establish and maintain effective working relationships with other employees and the public.
- Ability to work under pressure, communicate and present information.
- Ability to read, interpret, and apply clinic policies and procedures.
- Ability to identify problems, recommend solutions, organize and analyze information.
- Ability to establish priorities and coordinate work activities.
- Exposure to electronic health record preferred.
- Ability to work independently, be goal-directed and have strong organizational skills.
- Effectively multitask without compromising quality.
- Ability to comprehend and excel in both verbal and written communication, including proper telephone etiquette, face-to-face interactions, and electronic communications.
- Ability to communicate with individuals and small groups with credibility and confidence.
- Ability to handle difficult situations, remain calm under stress, manage emotional situations, display empathy and maintain positive communication during a rapidly changing/dynamic environment.
- Turn problems into opportunities by developing innovative and creative solutions.
- Demonstrate a friendly, positive attitude, display energy and drive in performing daily responsibilities.

- Must be flexible as well as easily adapt to a changing work environment which will require ongoing maintenance of job-related skills/activities.
- Must be willing to adjust work schedules in response to department or clinical needs.
- Able to manage and prioritize tasks simultaneously while working directly with patients who may exhibit diverse needs.

Equipment Operated:

- Standard office equipment including computers, fax machines, copiers, printers, telephones, etc.

Work Environment:

- Position is in a well-lit office environment. Occasional evening and weekend work.

Mental/Physical Requirements:

- Involves sitting approximately 90 percent of the day, walking or standing the remainder.
- Combination of sitting, standing, bending, light lifting and walking.
- Requires a full range of body motion including manual and finger dexterity and hand-eye coordination.
- Requires corrected vision and hearing to a normal range.
- Requires the ability to manage stressful situations.
- Occasional stress from varying demands.

Disclaimer: This description is intended to provide only basic guidelines for meeting job requirements. Responsibilities, knowledge, skills, abilities and working conditions may change as needs of the organization evolve.

Appendix B:
Sample Interview Questions

These are specific behavior-based questions for the different roles in patient access. Build on these to obtain the information needed to determine if the candidate has the skillset and abilities to address some of these common issues.

Standard Questions for Revenue Cycle Positions

There are many specific questions for each job title; this is a sampling of questions that could work for the job titles in this category.

- How do you handle conflict in the workplace? Have you had situations in your past when you disagreed with your supervisor and how did you handle it?
- Do you have an elevator pitch?
- What's the biggest challenge in your role?
- Tell me about a time when you weren't successful in providing good customer service. What did you learn and what would you do differently?
- How do you know when you've been successful in your role?
- How do you explain what you do to a 5-year old?

- You're talking with a coworker/patient/customer and you notice a mistake on your materials. How do you handle this? What do you say?
- Tell me about a time when you've made decisions and afterward regretted it.

Specific Questions for Revenue Cycle Positions

- Reimbursement Specialist
  - How do you manage all of the pulling and pushing that goes on within a practice?
  - Tell me about how you handle conflict with the practice owner or physicians.
  - How do you stay up to date on new reimbursement models?
  - Do you work with an outside firm for auditing? How has that worked in the past for you?
  - How do you keep up with the payor changes?
  - How are the fee schedules determined and audited?
- Medical Billing/Coding Specialist
  - How do you stay up to date on new requirements and coding information?
  - Walk me through your background and what makes this role enticing
  - Tell me about how you handle conflict with the management team.
  - Tell me about your past successes that you're proud of in your past roles
  - Which procedures have you most often billed in your current and prior positions?
  - Tell me about which practice management systems you have used? What did you like about them? Dislike?
  - How would you handle a situation that an account cannot be billed because the charting had never been completed?

- Financial Analyst
  - How would you present your data and reports to executives and higher-ups?
- Billing Office Supervisor
  - Why do you want to work in the revenue cycle department?
  - Tell me about which practice management systems you have used? What did you like about them? Dislike?
- Front Desk Clerk
  - How do you handle a patient who cannot pay the copay at time of visit?
  - How do you see your role as part of patient care?
  - Tell me about which practice management systems you have used? What did you like about them? Dislike?
  - What systems have you used for eligibility?
  - Let's role play a collections call. I will be the patient that owes $150.
- Coder
  - Tell me what you know about ICD-10 and CPT coding systems.
  - What CAC programs have you used?
  - What was the most difficult part transitioning to ICD-10?
- Office Manager
  - How would you describe the practice revenue cycle to a provider?
  - What do you know about MIPS?
  - Tell me your worse experience with the credentialing process.
  - What do you consider an acceptable A/R for a practice this size?

- Follow up Specialist
  - Tell me about a time that you didn't get the answer you wanted for a pre-authorization. What did you do to overturn the payor's decision?
  - Tell me about the process you use to appeal a claim.
  - What do you do if an insurance company wants to see the medical record prior to paying?

About the Authors

Penny M. Crow, MS, SHRM-SCP, RHIA, is a nationally recognized executive with progressive senior leadership experience in a wide range of healthcare organizations. As an RHIA, she has a successful track record in health information management, revenue cycle, risk management and quality improvement. Her MS in I-O Psychology, has fueled her passion about working with leaders to develop strategic thinking skills.

Christine Kalish, MBA, CMPE, is a senior executive and trusted healthcare advisor with deep experience in ambulatory care and academic medicine. She is a thought leader and strategist for emerging and expanding healthcare organizations. For more than thirty years, Kalish has been leading organizations and teams to develop critical infrastructure and growth planning to improve operations, workflow, human resources and revenue cycle. She continually searches for innovative ways to assist her clients so they can deliver quality care for the populations they serve.

Sharon Z. Ginchansky, MAOM, is a consultant specializing in leadership and organizational change. Her career spans more than twenty-five years of operational and human resources experience working as an executive in the healthcare field.

Contributor: Summer Humphreys, MBA